PRINCESS SPIDER
True Experiences of a Dominatrix

PRINCESS SPIDER
True Experiences of a Dominatrix

Princess Spider

First published in 2006 by
Virgin Books
Thames Wharf Studios
Rainville Rd
London W6 9HA

ISBN 0 7535 1039 1
ISBN 978 0 7535 10391

Typesetting by Phoenix Photosetting, Chatham, Kent

Printed and bound by
Bookmarque Ltd, Croydon, Surrey

*For my Father, my sons,
and all those who have served me.*

Some names have been changed to protect identities.

'Life, the universe
And everything, but for me
You are the answer'
Slave Mouse

'A slave cannot expect anything,
but can hope for everything'
Slave Daphne

CHAPTER ONE: THE SPIDER HATCHES

'When you see a spider, you get goosepimples. Or a jolt of fear, or an outright phobic reaction.'

Princess Spider

THE PRINCESS SPIDER OATH

You must recite your Oaths each morning. You will soon be instructed to assemble your own Altar of Respect.

I will serve and obey Princess Spider.
Each day I will lay down my loyalty to Princess Spider.
I will worship only Princess Spider.
I belong to Princess Spider.
I love Princess Spider.
My life is not my own.
My life is not my own.

I sit in my bondage throne – the spider at the heart of her web – and compose myself. Energy, nervousness, the spike of adrenaline, all of it could ruin my aim and send the session into a dark place where I would not want to follow. I breathe deeply, eyes closed, and focus. I offer a little prayer for the power I need. There is music, there are soft lights, there is incense. I feel the soft leather encasing my breasts and my bottom. The boots that embrace my legs. The ancient tools of torture are arranged around me in the dungeon. There are the silk-lined cages, a medieval rack, display cases filled with glittering arcane instruments, the 'dentist's' chair with its ecstasy of rubber hoses and masks hanging in a steel crook like some hideous octopus. Butt plugs and dildos stand erect in brutal black rubber. A St Andrew's cross, winches, pulleys, straps and hooks. Any and all variations of pain, degradation and humiliation. And the weaponry. An arsenal to reduce any man or woman. Floggers, canes, whips. Just to look at them is to be defeated. All of them known to my hands as intimately as if they were natural extensions of my arms, as if they were a part of me at my birth. This is my country of the damned. This is my dark unfettered world. I am at home. I find a zone of peace and concentration. I am ready.

The timid knock at the door. A voice calls out to enter, a powerful voice cut with danger and seduction. It is a mild shock to realise that voice is my own. Slave Twin enters on all fours, his eyes closed, his head bowed, subjugation made flesh. He wears a pair of briefs, a length of thin red rope coiled into the waistband. His scarred back is healing nicely. I ask him for the things he must bring to me. His journal. His chain. These things he has left in his car. Has he done this to test me? Or does he desire punishment? If so, he will get it. I will take the shape of his desire and turn it into something that savages him. I will blunt his sharp edges.

'Go and fetch them,' I purr. 'Hurry up!'

He eventually returns with a chain around his neck. I demand he kowtows before me. I allow him to kiss my boots. I demand he lights my cigarette. I allow him a sip of water. Time congeals around us. It is just him and me. Everything else is blurred. There could be someone in the room witnessing this and I would not be aware. I am the spider, and my prey is here.

'Any confessions for me today?' I ask.

He mumbles his reply, a wish he had that morning, a vision of rubbing his penis against my bottom.

Slowly, deliberately, I say: 'Cock inspection.'

He kneels and presents himself to me. This is his mistake. I kick him swiftly between the legs and he moans, threatens to crumple.

'Kneel!' I bark. He remains in position, trembling. I am training him well. I order him to tie the red rope to his balls. I tie the other end to a restraining pole in the centre of the dungeon. I force him down on all fours. Good dog. It is time.

I blindfold him. I let him hear me move around the dungeon. I put on my belt with its jangling attachments. I let him hear me withdraw a weapon from that beautiful savage collection. I shake out the leather tails of the flogger. I see his ears straining. The need to know what comes next, the delicious uncertainty.

I thrash his back and balls, pulling on the leash to drag his swollen genitals between his thighs and into my range. I ignore his gasps and groans. *This is what you want, this is what you get.*

Now for the cane. A few practice swings to warm me up and improve its flexibility. And to let him hear its song in the air, to know what flavour of pain to next expect. His thighs and buttocks grow taut. I beat him until he is rocking from side to side on his knees, flinching from the bite of the wood. And then, gently: 'Are you all right?'

'Yes, Mistress.' His voice is thick with desire.

I move close and stroke his violated flesh. The tenderness of my touch is almost as shocking to him. He twitches again. The confusion in his mind has taken him to the edge of his own levels of tolerance. He is mine to break.

I bring the steel back to my voice. 'On to the kneeling bench!'

He gingerly positions himself on all fours. Again with the cane. Accelerating, a new level of control, upping the ante to the extent that the pain becomes a part of him and then something *outside* of him. The pain connects us. It swarms around us, binding itself to every corner of the dungeon. The lights seem to flare as if feeding off the emotion. The cane grows warm to the touch. It slices the air. The speed grows to a point where its music is like that of a helicopter. Twin is statue hard, the cords in his arms and legs standing out. Sweat gleams against our skin. The cane breaks.

I step back, out of the moment. Clarity descends. I force him to stand in front of the pole and bind him fast to it. His head jerks around in an attempt to orient himself, trying to drink in any sliver of light to let him see what is coming next.

I have always loved candles. Their soft light turns skin to pale amber and picks out the glistening of eyes and mouths. Its play along the lengths of steel is something like magic. The flame dances as the breath of my prey becomes more ragged. The candles measure time in the way the wax wilts, melts, drops to the floor. Like the slaves themselves.

I pour molten wax across Twin's shoulders, back and buttocks. He arches and bucks, trying to dance his body away from the liquid fingers as they scrape a path across his flesh. I ask Twin how many strokes of the cane he has coming to him.

'I am owed ten thousand, seven hundred and seventy,' he whispers. I ask him what he could have done to build up such an account. How naughty has he been. How very, very naughty.

I ask him, 'How many mistresses have you served in the past?'

A beat. 'None like you, Mistress.'

It's not the correct answer, but I like it. 'None with my aroma?' I suggest, and take off my pink knickers, the ones he likes, and trawl them across his face. His bound cock twitches in appreciation. I attach clamps to his nipples. The chain hangs lightly between them. 'Weights?' I ask him.

'If Mistress wishes it.'

I pull lightly on the chain and his nipples spring erect. He shows me his teeth.

More wax. To keep him on his toes. I like to busk it, to throw a little spice into the mix when it's not really needed. It's like jazz: unpredictable, fluid, rhythmic. He is moving against the spatter of wax so violently that the animal print rug under his feet is sliding away, threatening to spill him to the floor. 'Pathetic!' I shriek at him. 'Stop sliding around. Did I ask you to dance yet?'

He becomes still and I lean in against his hot body. He feels the leather of my skirt, the cold dimpling of studs from my spank belt against his taut gut. 'I don't care about dancing with wax,' I tell him. 'I like to punish you.' I move to the incense holder and remove one of the sticks, breathe lightly on its smouldering end to enrage its coal. I dab this against Twin's testicles and he reacts as if electrocuted. In his cry is a sliver of untrammelled joy.

This slave. This Twin. He's a Body Slave of mine. A man granted special permissions within the world of domination. I allow him to serve me intimately. I grant him pussy worship. He is, after all, begging to serve his mistress. But he is not obedient. He does not stop when I tell him. He does not kowtow. He needs more training.

'Shall I sack you and find someone to fill your shoes? I will if I am not satisfied with you.' I'm teasing him. Am I teasing him? Let him leave with that question turning in his thoughts.

I lift the blindfold. I stroke his back, his buttocks. Wax falls away from him in translucent white fragments, like pieces of broken angels' wings. I release him. The session is over. I sit back in the throne and gather my thoughts. The music brings me down. My breathing returns to normal. My heartbeat slows. It has been a good session. He will not forget me lightly after that. I will be in his thoughts for hours.

Princesses are always waiting to be queen. I don't want to be a queen. I've never thought about promotion. I've always been called Princess through my life one way or another. When the name Princess Spider was first mentioned, it seemed to fit. It was poetic. Gentle, good, kind, yet with this dark attachment. It reflected my black and white character. I have a caring side ... and a reputation for being terribly cruel.

I receive an email from a guy called Roberts, my first client. He'd seen my picture on the website, liked it, and decided he desperately wanted to see me. He lived in Chiswick so I arranged to meet him there. It was strange to think that I could have bumped into him at any time wearing my smart two-piece suit because that's where I worked. He told me that he would be wearing a cream-coloured mac and I thought, here we go, I'm going to have a right perv on my hands. But I meet him and he's old. Really old. He's 86. My first client, standing sweating in his mac in the sweltering heat of high summer. And I'm thinking, heart attack, stroke, something's going to get him before we get back to the dungeon.

I said, 'The dungeon's in Mile End – will you be all right because you've got your mac on and it will be hot on the tube.'

He replied, 'I've got to keep my mac on because underneath it I'm wearing a chastity device and my TV training clothes.'

It's been a short journey, but I've come a long way. It's hard to believe I had a life so very different to this one just seven years ago. I was in a difficult relationship in the Midlands, where I was raised. Things were getting violent. I used to talk about it to a group of girls I 'met' in an internet chat room. I liked the anonymity at first, and the sense of community. You can open up to people more easily when you can't see them ... maybe there's some connection with blindfolds there! We talked about BDSM and played games with each other on the net.

Eventually I gathered up enough courage to come down to London and visit them. I ended up falling for one of them, Lisa, an Italian doctor. It was a heady time. She asked me to move down with my kids. It would mean a better life. It would mean being away from a woman who might cause me a serious injury at some point along the line. It didn't take long for me to decide. I came down to London in December 1999. When I was settled in with Lisa I was introduced to some of her friends. One of them was called Simone, a transsexual, whose wife worked at a West London Housing Association. It was a contact that got me my first job in the capital. Receptionist. You wouldn't believe this leather-clad woman of darkness started out sitting behind a desk being polite to people phoning up to rant about the state of their homes.

I realised I had to be quite stern in my day job. I was from a care background, having worked in the voluntary sector, and the company was finance driven. I went in with this very soft attitude: if someone called up to say their bath needed replacing, I'd say, hey, I'm ordering you the best one. My supervisor pulled me up and told me it was all about money. 'I know you care,' he said, 'but you've got to give them the bog standard.'

With Roberts, bumbling along on this tube until we arrive at Bank, where we had to catch a connecting train. And he said, 'Mistress, I've actually got my collar and lead on underneath this,' and he undid his tie, pulled his shirt open and there's this big collar and lead. He said, 'Would you do me the honour of leading me through the tube station? Could I please beg for this?'

And I thought, *what the hell, let's just go for it*. So I get this lead and I'm dragging this poor guy – in my smart work suit – and all these people are looking and I'd forgotten the security cameras and I thought someone was going to arrest us. But somehow we finally get to the dungeon. The lift's not working. Graham, the guy I'm living with, lives on the fourth floor, and by now it's really hot. I finally get him upstairs and sit him in the dungeon while I go off to get him a glass of water. Graham asked me if I'd got Roberts with me, and I said, 'Yes, but he's pretty old, I think he's going to die.'

I put him in the dungeon and got him some water and Graham put his head around the door and mouthed to me, 'My God, he really is old.'

Roberts, a real gentleman, politely handed me my tribute in

a white envelope. And he said, 'What would you like as a gift?'

This threw me as I didn't realise that gifts were a part of the deal. But he was sitting there in his TV gear and it reminded me that my telly was on the blink so I thought, I'll have a TV. We were pissing ourselves because he was saying I'll buy you a TV and he *was* a TV.

He basically just wanted gentle play, worshipping boots, things like that. I had some stuff at Graham's, things he'd kindly bought for me, and I had some great boots, they were knee high, black with a black heel and a steel tip. They zipped up at the side but they had intricate D-rings up the back that glinted when I turned my leg this way and that. I wore it with a little PVC skirt and a black top. It was all soft and shiny and sleek and shimmery. The smell of leather filled the room. I saw Roberts swallow, lick his lips.

I learned very quickly how to speak to people in my office job, how to close a conversation if time was getting on. How to control a conversation. I carried this skill over to the slave world. I was popular at work because people would come in steaming about their troubles and I'd say: 'Sit down, give me your details, would you like a cup of tea while you're waiting?' and in this way I'd disarm them. In the end people would call up and ask to speak to me.

I lived in South London when I relocated to the capital. I noticed pretty quickly that everyone around me was quite snappily dressed. I realised I'd need to get hold of some clothes if I wasn't going to get a reputation for being grungy. Simone bought me lots of gear, including fetish gear, vibrators, all this stuff I'd never even seen before, let alone held in my hands. We celebrated by going to a fetish club called The Fringe, run by a guy called Master Keith, who is now a good friend. I didn't have any high heels at this point, so I had to borrow them from a neighbour.

I've still got the outfit. PVC top, little black skirt with a chain on, black stockings and borrowed black stilettos. I felt powerful in those clothes. I've always felt a powerful person, but those clothes enhanced it, gave me a stature that had somehow always been there, but needed just the right gear to draw it out of me. I felt like a different person.

The club was amazing, a life-changing experience. Simone asked me to spank her while we were there. I'd never spanked anyone in public before. I was nervous, but also a little curious. And turned on. So Simone got comfortable and I started spanking away at her, and before long someone else came up and asked me if I'd do the same to them, and I thought: 'Oh, this sounds good. This feels good to me.' It felt as if a switch had been thrown. I had found something that felt utterly right, utterly me. I knew it was as much to do with how I must look, the power and mystique, as well as the erotic slap of a hand as it paddles a nice little portion of firm female flesh.

Later, when things had calmed down a bit, Simone said to me, 'Did you know there are professional dominatrices?'

I was stunned. I said, 'No, I didn't know that.'

'Oh yeah, they earn tons of money. You can make a living at this kind of thing. You were really good – I mean, look at the way you handled those guys.'

So that was it. A door had opened to me. I was standing on the threshold looking in at a world that was at once the most alien and yet the most recognisable thing I'd ever seen. I wanted to know more. Lots more. I wanted to shut the door behind me on my old life and immerse myself in whatever the new world had to offer. I wanted to lock that door for good.

'Do you like what you see?' I asked Roberts.

'Yes, Mistress.'

'Would you like a closer look?'

'Yes please, Mistress.'

I lifted one foot and slowly, deliberately placed it between his legs, making sure I lightly pinched a little of the skin of his thigh. He gasped.

'Would you like to kiss my boot?' I asked him.

'I would like nothing better, Mistress,' he said. His voice was ragged now, and I could see his pulse in his neck. His face had turned red. I asked him if he was all right, if he would like some more water, but he assured me he was fine.

He courteously cupped my heel with one hand as he raised my boot to his mouth. He knew what he was doing. He was a class act. He ran his lips and tongue over the polished leather, inhaling deeply as if trying to suck the smell of my feet through the impenetrable hide. I stroked his head and let him fondle my boots for as long as he wanted.

He just totally loved it. He was one of the first to say I was too pretty to be a mistress. A lot of people say that. Why are you a mistress, you're too pretty? And I say I like being a mistress. I like the lifestyle.

So he was my first one. He was a sweet old man.

The excitement was intense, walking into work the next day realising my new future was unfolding, like the petals of a rose. My director found out about it but he was great. He knew I was writing fetish poetry and stories in my lunch break and planned to go, as he put it, 'spanking' in the evenings. It was great, a real vibrant buzz. In a short time I had moved from hotel work at Gatwick and Heathrow and the Thistle at Marble Arch to a real dungeon. I was on cloud nine, and the money was fantastic.

I was on my way.

PERMISSION TO SPEAK: Gary

'I met Princess Spider when she moved into the flat where I live in South London. I've known her for around seven years. We went on a few dates, got together, we had a little bit of an intimate relationship, but it was always quite casual. We had some good times. We're great friends now. I'm really happy for her, what she's doing now. Some people may look at that life

and think it's a bit odd, they might have their own views and opinions on it, but the more fun in life the better, as far as I'm concerned. She's always been ambitious. She's very intelligent, knows what she wants and how to go about getting it.

'I thought she was lovely, charming, quite funny. She's got the X factor. Something special about her, she's got like an aura that attracts people to her. The fact that she has a different lifestyle is attractive too. People don't feel threatened or insecure around her. Her confidence rubs off on you. She also has a deeply mature side to her as well.

'I'd always been curious about the social side of BDSM but never known how to get through the door. So she invited me to a few of her parties. It's not really my scene, but it was an eye-opener.

'So now I've been to a few of these parties and you get all kinds of people. Extremely well-bred types, very successful. Any background whatsoever. Judges, doctors, lawyers, down to the average Joe Bloggs. Quite artistic to my eye. Creative, sexual, a weird mixture of costumes, characters. Nobody's taking any notice of anybody else. It's a very friendly atmosphere. What's going on around you is extremely surreal. I'm not into it, so I don't have any special costumes, but I wore a pair of satiny trousers, black boots, a black vest and a long leather jacket. One party was at quite a small place in Tulse Hill. I was like an escort for her. There was nowhere to hide. I was just amazed at what was going on. The scenery was different from one room to another. A cave atmosphere, to an old-fashioned traditional gentlemen's club, then you've got someone naked in a corner doing things to himself, and someone chained up getting whipped, and a couple having sex. It's just so bizarre.

'I'm quite straitlaced. I can't be manipulated. Nothing fazes me. We've got a normal relationship so she doesn't play any games with me. It wouldn't work, really. I think she likes me because I'm the opposite. She probably saw me as a challenge but it didn't get to that stage. I'm pretty strong-minded. I won't change. But our relationship didn't really last long enough for *anything like that to develop. I find it funny, rather than take it seriously, when she says, "I'm going to whip you if you don't get a move on." It's a bit more light-hearted.'*

Before all this happened, I had my palm read. I believe in fate. I believe that our lives are mapped out for us to a greater or lesser degree. How you follow that route, how you make fate work for you, is where you succeed or fail. I have dreams that come true although I never saw anything to do with domination in dreams. The last time I had my palm read, I wasn't sure where my relationship was going. I was seeing a doctor and she was training, so even me with all my charisma and charm … I knew that might not be enough to keep her – and I didn't want to hold her back. This woman said I would meet a knight and he would change my life. Well I don't know about knights, but I met Twin, who's a chief's son from Nigeria.

The first thing I saw at that party at The Fringe that was really amazing was Master Keith and his girlfriend. He'd tied her to this great big hoist and wrapped her body in lots of ropes. Her breasts had been squeezed through two small holes and were sticking out, swollen and tight. He was fucking her with this huge aubergine and I was rubbing my eyes, saying to Simone, 'I can't believe I'm seeing this.'

And she said, 'Don't worry about her, he's a very good master, he knows all about safe words and that kind of thing.'

Safe words – that was the first time I'd come across that term. I decided to do some research so I put a few of the trigger words I'd heard into a search engine and slowly built up this strange dossier all about BDSM. I was impatient. I wanted to be a part of things. So Lisa helped me. She took some pictures of me in a lot of sexy gear at her house, I created a Yahoo! profile, put my kinky information on along with my mobile phone number, and some of the photos, and went live. That's how people first contacted me.

I'd go to the office in the daytime, deal with hundreds of frantic calls a day – 'Hello, Housing Association, can I help you?' – that sort of thing, and then I'd nip away from my desk at break times and call the guys back, having to switch to this mysterious woman with the commanding teasing sensual voice. It was bizarre.

I used to write fetish stories in my breaks. I printed one out for my director who I really fancied – he gave me five interviews before he gave me that job. I had a feeling he'd give it to me after the first interview, but he really liked talking to me.

He said, 'You're wasting your time here, you should be doing something more creative.'

Graham was the guy I met after the thing with Lisa fizzled out. He was into BDSM too and actually had a dungeon in his flat. His whole flat contained things related to that whole scene. I thought it had a really nice vibe, it seemed like a very comfortable place to live. There were all these things there that I'd never seen before. Leather hoods, punishment equipment, chains and whips.

He had built an imaginary world around his obsession and had called it Silk Planet. He had constructed a website around it and used it as a way of enticing slaves to send presents to the mistresses. I became one of them. He said to me, 'I've got this character in mind called Princess Spider. Why don't you take her name?'

I was touched, and excited. Nobody had ever named me before. He dressed me in a black leather skirt, leather shirt, leather cap and slid a bowie knife into my belt.

Graham took one look at me and said, 'Oh my God, it's you.'

He took some photographs. That was where Princess Spider's image was born. That's her look. I was the right height and build for his creation. But there was more than that going on. I felt as though the character had always been waiting for me to step into it, like a forgotten suit of clothes hanging in a wardrobe. I felt completely comfortable, and inspired, when I dressed as Princess Spider for the first time. A part of me that I never knew existed pushed through and took control. But at the same time she was really familiar to me. I suppose Spider is a patchwork of personalities that I've built up over the years. She's a part of me, and an extension of me. And sometimes I never know what she's going to do. Which also means my slaves don't, either. A good thing, I think ...

Princess Spider developed when she was with Graham. I've never shaved a guy and he was getting me to shave his balls. I was thinking, *God, what if I cut him?* He liked to wear this hood with a cock attached to the mouthpiece. He asked me to straddle him, and I'm thinking *Hello, I've never sat on one of these before*. I was learning at the same time as actually doing it. It was the world I wanted and it was all exciting. The only boundaries within the fetish world involve your own imagination.

As a tutor, Graham was a great guy to learn from. We had some great fun too. We collaborated on a story called *The Future* that we incorporated in the Silk Planet website about cells where men were put away to await an operation that drained their sperm from them for genetic processing, to create a superior army of dominatrices. It was liberating to possess this character and give my imagination the chance to go where it wanted to. There were no rules, no restraints (not in that sense of the word, at least!) and no limits.

Graham was getting a lot of traffic at his site, but, helping him with admin and mailing tasks one day, I was sure we could improve it.

I said to him, 'You must have guys who don't do as you say. Or who call once and never again. Where's the reject list?'

He was a very organised guy and he pointed me in the direction of a row of files. There were hundreds of potential clients in there, people who saw an advert for Silk Planet, wanted to speak to a mistress but none were available, missed calls, and so on. One Saturday afternoon I sat down with the list and the phone and methodically went through them all, ringing them up. I had the stern but playful voice going, the lot: 'Hi, this is Princess Spider, why aren't you calling us any more?'

Later, having introduced a healthy injection of new clients, I noticed Graham smiling and lightly shaking his head.

'What?' I asked him.

He said: 'You're a natural.'

> I've had dreadlocks since 1994. I just wanted a change.
> A friend of mine was into Rasta men and she had lots of
> drawings. I was fascinated and wondered if I could do
> that to my hair, because it's naturally curly. I got the
> hairdresser to perm little dreadlocks into my curls. They
> were quite funky when they were short but I thought it
> made me appear too masculine. So I grew them. A
> friend of mine told me that when my dreadlocks grew
> long, my life would change. And she was right.

How do I define it, this sweet-sour acronym, this BDSM? The letters stand for Bondage Discipline Sado-Masochism.

Bondage is a side of things that doesn't really interest me too much, unless it's a form of mental bondage. I hate the time consumption of physically tying somebody up. It can look amazing, and aesthetically pleasing, to see all this rope and intricate knotting strategically positioned around a naked body, but it's not for me, especially if I only have an hour in a dungeon to dominate somebody. I prefer to restrict the mind. I think it's a far greater tool to use the brain than the rope. Mind control can prove your superiority more formidably than the wrapping of twine around a wrist or an ankle.

Discipline for me is about training men to become the respectful gentlemen that men used to be, like knights of old. All loyal slaves build an altar of respect, which should contain a figurine goddess and candles. They recite their mantras or oaths each day, or they use pictures of me by an ornate mirror and recite their vows. The shrine may just be a collection of images, or whatever they use to associate with me if they can't have my image on show, but it will be the centrepiece of their slave life.

Sadism is the sexual pleasure or gratification gained from the infliction of pain and suffering upon another person. I enjoy it very, very much; time has no boundary for me here. Some say I play on the dark side of BDSM, which means that I like to draw blood, like a black witch. I like needle play and have made slaves bleed on many occasions with my weapons, or my teeth. I do not see blood as a taboo subject within this lifestyle, although I accept that some do. My cruelty is legendary but so also is my compassion, that's why I have so many fans. I'm witty in session and my boys love the way I trip them up.

Most say I'm a white witch, however, because of my healing skills. Perhaps I'm both. Some say I'm like Obi-Wan Kenobi (a great tutor). I seem to fit several descriptions.

Masochism. All pain-loving slaves are the best to torment. Body slaves have to be strong and brave in this regard. This is why Twin is so-called. He is my soul-mate in pain. We play hard exploring all aspects of these dark arts. I'm happy to inflict severe physical or psychological pain as an expression of cruelty, a means of intimidation, deterrent or punishment, or as a tool for the extraction of information or confessions. It all sounds divine to me – I love it! I will put Body Slaves through the most severe torments, even if it means denying myself sexual pleasure or even seeing them. Because, in many ways, that's the best torment: not to torment at all. They all want it, crave it. But I might simply sit and drink tea and make idle chat while dressed in something provocative. It cracks them up.

All of my slaves have boundaries, but I will torment in any way their imagination and physical being will allow them. I care for them too. It's all a learning curve incorporating 'their pain, my pleasure'. I use that phrase a lot. Some slaves like to involve themselves in self-bondage while I'm away from them. Because self-bondage is performed alone, it carries a heightening of sensation, a frisson that comes as much because of an increased risk as anything else. Someone who is able to tie themselves up well can cause themselves wild excitement, because the danger is enhanced.

PERMISSION TO SPEAK: Slave Twin

'I believe to a certain extent that BDSM can improve you as a person psychologically. It can strengthen you, prepare you for certain situations in life. But it can also be detrimental. It's all about the psychology of where you are, how strong you are at the start, your character. Like drugs or alcohol. It can be your nemesis. If you're happy with it, it can make you. I'm half black, half white. My mother was Scottish, my father from Nigeria. I believe I have an insight into both cultures. I transcend both of them. I'm happy with my deviancy. As long as I don't hurt anybody, then it's fine. I would never want to be a person who would torture somebody for information. That is an abomination for me. It's purely within a playful framework that I want to use it.

'Pain is an interesting concept. It fascinates me that you can build up a resistance to it. Your imagination is great in that respect. You say yeah, I can take it. But the reality is that you have to bring that back. I have had a lot of straight relationships. I have a lot of straight thoughts that don't include BDSM influences. I chose to explore it more. I experimented before I immersed myself in the scene, so I had a vague idea of how much I could take. But I have never been to a mistress, unless they've been quite bad, who took you straight into an extreme level. First they want to know what you can take. They very rarely go into a hard session from the word go, even if you say you want it. It's all relative. I've said I want a hard session and they've come in a little too hard. You have to build up a level of trust between yourself and the mistress. They have to get to know you, and understand what you're looking for. That happened with me. She knew I was open to new experiences, but she also took me into new territory. Slowly, helping me to understand my own limits and then stretch myself.

'One incident I wasn't really into was a severe restraint. I was bound and gagged. I didn't like it. It became too much for me and I passed out. At the point I was getting dizzy and said that I wasn't feeling too good, that gave me a lot of confidence in her because she immediately released me, gave me water and looked after me. From then on I was able to go further because I was utterly confident that she would do the right thing, the smallest signal and she would release me. Subsequently I was able to go a lot further with her because I no longer had the fear stifling me. It's the fear of pain that makes it more painful. Once you're relaxed you can take more. You need to find a zone where you can deal with it and absorb it. Once you're with someone you have confidence in you can begin to extend your boundaries and learn about yourself. I believe the whole concept of pain, within S and M, to be not all that different from anything else in the world. I used to play rugby and you go through a lot of pain purposefully in rugby, hitting, getting hit, you get up and you get a buzz out of it. Give me what you've got and I'll deal with it. I don't think the S and M pain is necessarily a greater pain, maybe it's more ritualised and direct, but in terms of what you can take and be prepared to take, it's not so different. If I was a soldier and I was captured and threatened with torture I'd say, "Listen, let me write everything down for you." As I look at it, I couldn't survive that. It's a totally different thing. It's a sexual thing for me. Even if you don't get excited directly sexually, there's definitely some level of sexual trade-off.'

Another early session involved a home visit. I was nervous about this because it was the first time I had ever gone to a client's house and there was an element of danger involved, although I had seen the slave in the dungeon on a number of occasions and felt an affinity with him, even to the point of deciding that he was worthy of becoming a Body Slave.

I left instructions with a friend as to where I was going, and informed my client that I had done so. I arrived at his house in the south of London a little before seven p.m. I collected my tribute – a substantial one, considering the time I was giving to him – in the customary white envelope, and allowed myself to be ushered through to the living room. It was to be the last order I took from him for the next twelve hours.

We had dinner and I relaxed. I know people, I can suss them out pretty quickly, and I knew this session would be all right. We had a night of inventive, enjoyable play and got to know each other even better. I informed him that he would become my Body Slave, my first, and we slept together in the same bed, but only after I had placed him at the end, and secured him in a tight knot . . .

Princess Spider woke. Her Body Slave lay at the foot of the ornate cast-iron bed. He had been locked into sleep the previous night and, tightly bound, was unable to stir.

Mistress lay there for a while running her leather-gloved hands through her golden hair, running her fingertips over her black silkily seamed stocking tops. She smiled and adjusted her position.

She kicked her Body Slave and lit a cigar.

'Slut, wake up, clean my pussy now! It's almost time to milk you.'

Slave Benson looked up at the clock, its ticking silver hands read 6.30 a.m. 'Yes, Mistress.'

Clumsily turning towards his Goddess, he placed his head between Mistress's thighs.

Mistress spread herself, closing her eyes and lazily smoking her cigar. She placed her purple riding crop against his shoulder blades.

'Just in case you get your rhythm wrong,' she warned. Laughing, she thrashed him with the crop. It bit into his flesh three times. Her pale flesh was so inviting, her vanilla aroma caressing him. There would be compassion, but only until Mistress climaxed.

Writhing around on the front of his leather hood, Mistress ordered him to suck harder on her clitoris. Slave Benson's pace increased, his penis was throbbing out of control. He feared he might climax alongside her before officially being ordered to.

His cock-sheath clenching his swollen penis, he knew he had to hang on.

Mistress's silver high heels dug into his flesh as she rode the ripples of her eclipse.

She cropped her slave again as her orgasm rose to its shattering peak. Mistress's metronomic strokes tore into his morning flesh.

She slid off her leather gloves. Mistress ordered Slave Benson to stroke his penis.

'Wank for me, you reject. Into your jerk jar.'

'Yes, Mistress. I aim to please only you.' Mistress's regime was tough and he realised he was being tested. Hands firmly around his erection, he obeyed and chanted his Mistress Prayer:

'I am the lowliest of creatures in thy realm. Thy chattel who serves thee and worships thee loyally and faithfully beg thee, my magnificent Goddess. I beg that by my servitude I may be judged worthy. My mere existence in thy magnificent presence is a crime for I am mindless, inferior and undeserving of thee. If it so pleases thee I willingly submit myself to be painfully cleansed for my crimes against thee. I beg for mercy although I deserve no mercy and expect no mercy.'

Her appetite was insatiable.

His climax was imminent. His panting breath Mistress found amusing. She closely watched his climax and raised her crop once more to finish his fantasy with a sharp overpowering volley across his back and buttocks.

Mistress released him. The slave had stepped inside his mistress's web and he almost cried at the power and wonder that was around him.

The main reason for deciding to go pro-Domme was because of my children. When I first got here I couldn't get them in to school for three months. I had to buy all their books and the uniforms ... my wages couldn't cope with the demand so I had to borrow money. I wanted to be independent, and to be in a position to be able to give them something, the things in life that I never had. I was earning around £25K by January 2001, the dommeing supplementing my £17.5K wage. My children are my driving force. I want to leave something for them.

What I do in my life is really no different to many relationships, it's just a little more extreme, there's a little more play involved. It's a codified activity. In houses up and down the country sub/dom relationships occur naturally. One person takes charge, the other is more deferential. It's how relationships work. If you have two headstrong people butting up against each other over things, arguments break out. There has to be a little give and take in relationships. Give and take is what BDSM is all about. It's a perfect symbiosis. The bond between a mistress and her slaves is incredibly strong.

Who among us has never tied a lover up with silk scarves on a bed, or playfully smacked a naked bottom as a lover walks past, damp from the shower? When does this become erotic bondage? When is it spanking? Isn't it always these things? Don't the lines become blurred, the semantics faintly ridiculous? Is it all done to protect ourselves from the truth, that, at heart, we all like a little slap and tickle, whether dressed in a PVC gimp suit or not? Aren't we all a little kinky? A little perverse? What's wrong with taking the less than ordinary approach; being naughty, but nice?

With paying clients I sometimes get sexually aroused but satisfy myself when I get home to my partner. I get more mental stimulation from a session, really. The first session with any slave is always fantastic for me, I mould them into a submissive bundle, and in many cases it improves their sex lives and their relationships with their partners. It's a form of therapy in many ways, and I do meet clients who have a more conventional psychotherapist. Sessions with me work in tandem and work well. A lot of therapists who have become aware of me have encouraged clients to continue with their sessions because it helps them. I listen to their problems, and many have erectile dysfunction problems. I can help them with this and advise them of what to think. All those naughty thoughts we keep locked away, I encourage them to bring them to the fore. I have never really been shocked by what I have heard, but I can see what they describe, visually and mentally. Some men shake before me. I enjoy their nervousness, feed off it, and I coach them to be more confident.

My most recent new boy, Slave Alice, has no kneecap in one leg. I told him to sit, not kneel, before me. He was grateful for this and I think it helped him to relax with me. I guessed he had a strong feminine side to him, and I was right. He willingly explored stockings, but he was afraid, because he told me his legs were not fit for my eyes (he had many scars). But I encouraged him. Stockings were the logical answer; they would cover his legs and give him confidence. He loved it and walked quite contentedly around the dungeon. I believe this is one of my strengths, to see very quickly the problems to be solved, and to turn them around so that they almost become advantages. Anyway, Alice had a great first session and he will see me again. It's great to find new slaves who you know you've flicked a switch with.

I can get very turned on during a session, but it's usually because of what we're doing, and the atmosphere and the environment, as opposed to the client alone. Sometimes they can be a complete dish, but very boring to talk to. I like interesting men and most are, I have found. I hate strong body odour and I will tell men off for that.

My figure is not what it was. I'm no longer 38-24-38. I'm more 38-29-42! So is body shape still important? There is a saying that big girls have more fun, I could say yes, damn right we do! I know I have a good mind and I care, I love; men flock around me still and love chatting to me. It amuses me and makes me feel very loved. Does this take up my time? Well yes, but hey, I'm here for the third time so I'll make the most of it. At the moment I have Rooster, Master Peter, Master Simon, my old chauffer Norman, and Mistress Raven all contacting me for dates. Isn't it madness?

CHAPTER TWO: SECRET STRANGERS

'Princess Spider can do anything she likes because she's a superior mistress. She can break balls and break the rules.'

Princess Spider

Control has its part to play in how I've shaped my life. Yes, I'm a fatalist, but there's much to be said about making your own fate, about carving out the channels beforehand, so the river of your life allows you to go with the flow. I like it that I decide the hours I work, the price I charge, the customers I take on. I don't have any arses to kiss (well, not in that way…), no office politics to worry about. I don't have to run for the bus or skip lunch because I'm too busy. I don't have reports to file or quotas to fill. I'm in charge. I answer to nobody.

Typical introductory email to Princess Spider:

I have looked at your contact page.

If I have served you well enough you may reward me as you see fit for my services. My likes are: chastity and bondage, I am very much into tight corsets, posture collars, high heels, butt plugs, breath play, leather, latex, PVC, plastic, and boot-licking. I am not into pain at all.

My job skills are very portable and if you accept me as your live-in slave I will have no problems finding a job once I am there if you wish me to have an outside job. I am an auto mechanic by trade and I have know-how in the fixing of households, be it painting, dry walling, plumbing etc. I have built all my own bondage equipment and if you wish could do some additions or upgrade your dungeon.

Thank you for reading my message. If you have any questions or want more details please contact me by email.

Your humble servant and rubber doll,

Darren

The slave is also the master, in a strange kind of way. It's like any other business. These are your customers, so you have to treat them well, otherwise they won't come again. It's important to respect them, to be attentive to their needs, their desires and their fantasies. It's no good steaming in with the cane on some new client if they don't like it, or if they prefer to be warmed up first with floggers, paddles and quirts. My slaves are dear to me. I care about them and it's nice to develop trust between you to a point where they can submit totally to you and they know there's nothing to worry about. Coming to me, for a lot of slaves, is like therapy. Better than therapy. We're like a big family.

But it's not just all about what *they* can take from a session. I like my fun too. I enjoy dominating slaves, but sometimes, if I allow it, I will grant them a little time in which to worship a part of my body of my choosing. Not every slave is allowed this access. To become a Body Slave is no easy task. You have to earn this privilege.

Slaves will buy magazines to select their mistresses. The old school will look for mistresses who wear leather. Leather gloves, leather cap, leather boots, all the traditional stuff that was around in the 1940s, '50s and '60s. They like that kind of thing. A time when ladies wore gloves a lot, nice stockings, fitted suits. That wholesome Doris Day image. The younger slave boys like mistresses who look tacky or sluttish, so they'll go for the PVC clothing. I'll wear PVC if a slave wants me to. I'm not going to put on leather just because I prefer it. If I didn't wear what he wanted then that's a potential client gone for good. It's like a dentist. There's no point filling the wrong tooth.

I sometimes wear '50s stuff when I'm going out. I like the way they dressed back then. I'm in no doubt that a lot of slaves' fetishes were inspired by their aunts or nannies or mothers holding their hands tight while wearing those pretty, close-fitting gloves. Parents were quite strict in those days too. As were the teachers in school; it was not unusual to find corporal punishment used on a daily basis. Bullying too was rife, not treated as seriously then as it is now.

Some slaves are mistress collectors. They could see me today, another mistress the next day, someone else next week. They just like different experiences with different mistresses. They don't have any loyalty. The slave boys who serve me once a month get collared and given a slave name. Once they have a name I can put them in my diary and know they'll be my regulars. If someone visits more than just once, they get a contract too, which basically says that I can do anything with them, and, if I allow it, they can do things with me. And they usually do come more than once ... unless I don't fit their fantasy.

I've had some wonderful presents over the years. Intriguing presents too. I have a bike that was given to me from a guy who worked in the media for the US Navy. He paid all my tributes with his US Navy credit card, which was probably a bit naughty but I wasn't going to complain.

I met him via an internet chat room. He was called Sailor Peter. He told me he was coming over to London, and that he was really interested in domination. His wife was suffering from MS and couldn't get about much. She was into it too but couldn't physically get involved anymore. Anyway, he liked my pictures on the internet. I was working in the office at the time.

My friend there came in with a flash American mountain bike. I had a go on it, really liked it, and when I got home I emailed Sailor Peter to tell him that I was interested in having such a bike and that they could be purchased at a certain chain store in the States. It was a great bike and I instructed him to buy it as part of my tribute. He got it flown over; it was a flat-pack job, something you have to put together yourself. I met him at the Thistle Hotel in Marble Arch and he'd constructed the bike in his room.

I was wearing blue iridescent jeans with a cropped top and a purple spangled jacket and flat shoes. I looked like a beautiful shiny insect. He opened the door and here was this big American naval guy, much bigger than me and I'm no weed. He said 'close your eyes', and I didn't really want to – he was only my second client in hotels and for a moment I thought he was going to put an axe in my head. But then he led me deeper into the room and told me to open my eyes and wow, this bike was there. I had a little go on it in the room. We went out and had some dinner and then I took him sight-seeing. I felt like an escort as well as a dominatrix, but I didn't mind. We had a lovely evening taking in all the famous London landmarks before returning to his room where I gave him a spanking session to remember. The following day we went to Marks & Spencer because he wanted to stock up on some food and clothes before he left. There was a really nice red suit on display and he pointed out that it would be a great colour for me. He persuaded me to try it on. It was a nice Italian-look office suit and boy, it fit like a glove. The reaction I got from all the guys outside the changing room waiting for their partners was awesome. Jaws dropping like flies. Sailor Peter said, in this lush American drawl, 'That's it, honey. You're having it.' He pulled out this Navy credit card and bought it for me.

My best gift is my Galatian's helmet. It's a replica, but it's the right size and weight – very heavy – I knew this guy, Mr Turnbull, was my Roman history guy and he's sent me various gifts. Books, DVDs, models of gladiators, all related to Roman history because he knows of my passion for military history, battle strategies, that kind of thing. I've still not met him.

The most astonishing instance of gift-buying I ever experienced was courtesy of Slave Benny in Bromley. I rang him and arranged to meet him. He saw me just the once. He took me shopping to this fabulous leather emporium and bought me a black leather cape with four or five inches of fox fur on the cuffs and collar. I can't remember how much it was exactly but it was around a grand. It looks really elegant. I thought that would be enough, but there was also this long smoky-grey mottled leather coat with square mother of pearl buttons. It had a thick rabbit fur collar. He bought me that as well, for 700 quid. He escorted me back to my house, said thank you for my time, and he left. He could have had any number of dungeon sessions with me for the amount he shelled out on those two coats ...

It's traditional to bring Mistress a tribute – a fee. It's called a tribute because originally dommes didn't work legally and didn't declare their earnings or pay tax. So if you say it's a tribute it's not technically a payment. I insist they bring the tribute in a white envelope. It's easier to put it in your bag. And if the Inland Revenue are watching, I'm totally legit. I'm squeaky clean. There aren't many that are, that's for sure.

The gift-buying thing is the slaves' way of displaying their affection for you, their willingness to serve. They want to please you. It's a bit like a birthday present, you give them a brief as to what kind of things you like and it's always interesting to see what they bring you as a gift. Martin, a South African slave, bought me a red leather jacket with black piping. It's beautiful. Most of my gifts have been personal things, rather than anything else. Most people bring me wine. The most practical gifts, such as stockings – I go through hundreds of pairs of stockings in a year – are a big help, even if they're the expensive ones. Well, a mistress has to look her best, doesn't she? It all adds up to a lot of money, and maintaining that quality look is difficult so you get your slaves to chip in. They're only too happy to help out. It gives them a real sense of pride and belonging to know that those dear French stockings, the one with the seam up the back that they've been allowed to tongue, have come out of their own pockets.

When I was starting up I thought it would be a good idea to get my clients to help me buy some of the toys to kit out my dungeon. That's another way forward, especially if you're lucky enough to have your own space, rather than a rented dungeon. It's important to be on the level with the slaves from the off. They know and you know that this is a business. They are paying for a service; you are charging to provide what they need. One of the first things we'll discuss is money. I know how long they've been saving up for sessions. I'll agree, if they're struggling, to a smaller tribute for less time, or time outside the dungeon, because obviously I'm having to pay to rent the dungeon.

I have a couple from Ireland who come over to see me on a regular basis. Money's no obstacle to them and they pay me what I'm worth. Actually, they pay more than anybody else. They want to do this. They bring booze and we'll drink in session because it's more a social thing with them. They bought me some leather thigh-high boots. But gifts can be anything, perfume, chocolates, flowers. I bought an X-box for my kids at the start of my career. A lot of money I earned at the start went on the kids. Expensive trainers, that kind of thing. This kind of work has presented me with the chance to give them things they wouldn't otherwise have.

Every slave must have a name. It's a way of sloughing off their everyday identity for a little while so that they can feel comfortable in an unusual environment. It helps promote the idea of a different world. And they are different people when they come to see me. They've shed their skins. They behave differently in my dungeon. The name helps them to forget who they really are and inhabit a fresh face for a little while.

The way I come up with their new names has a lot to do with how they look, but equally what their personality is like. Unless they've been named by a prior mistress, I can usually tell within five minutes of meeting them what the names I'm going to give them will be. They don't get a choice. It's Mistress's privilege. If they don't like it, tough. I'll tend to name the ones who are close to me and who I talk to quite a lot, and develop a rapport with. Mouse, for example, has got quite a rounded face, cute little ears, a skinhead and glasses. He looks like, well … a mouse. He shuffles about. I named Daphne because I detected a feminine side to his nature. We talked a lot about that, and it's something he's now exploring under my instruction. Benson I named because he was an old-school gentleman, with traits of a butler. Rooster because he henpecks. Dumpling contacted me after he saw the TV show. He wanted to be my slave. He's as tall as me but quite round, chubby but nice face. He is extremely polite. Twin because he's my soul-mate, my lover, my best friend.

They all help me out if I need them, if I'm arranging a stage show, for example. They'll all do their best for me and I can rely on them to be there when it matters.

They all open metaphorical doors for me to some lesser or greater degree. Mouse had a relationship with a female that went badly wrong. He decided he wanted to explore his gay side and I helped with that. I was bullied at school because I was involved in lesbian relationships. At the time it was very traumatic for me. It's more acceptable now than it was then, but there are still some extremely intolerant people around. I talked with Mouse about this. I said, 'You've got to be very strong because being a gay person is the most difficult path you can choose. Everybody will victimise you. It's more liberated than when I was 16, but it's still difficult for a gay man to get out there and be settled. You've got to make the right choice for the right reasons.'

The way he coped with that helped me to understand myself more. It's a symbiotic relationship, this business of mistress and slaves. We feed off each other. I'm not just there for the whackings and the waxings and the wankings. I'm a confidante sometimes. A mother figure. A crutch. I can be closer to these people sometimes than their own mothers, lovers or friends. The mistress offers a unique therapy that nobody else can provide.

PERMISSION TO SPEAK: Slave Twin

'I've been interested in BDSM as far back as I can remember. I came to the scene when I was about 19 or 20 when I came to live in London. One day I found a contact for a mistress. That was my first experience, and knowing that other people thought and felt the same way as I did empowered me. I expressed my obsession via my art. Long before I met anybody in the scene I had drawings that were my fantasies. Because I was able to draw I was able to take them further than most people might have. I was able to make them a reality in a way, through the drawings.

'I've searched for a trigger and I remember being at boarding school when I was nine or ten years old and having pre-sleep imaginings of powerful, developed sexual involvement. I haven't tried to psychoanalyse myself about it. My mother was a fairly powerful woman, so maybe it came from her. My father was quite strict, I had a fear of him, although throughout my life he never did anything to elicit that. But I always held him in awe. It was my mother who disciplined me. He was very cool – he'd just lecture me.

'I love how daydreams and fantasies can intertwine with reality where BDSM is concerned. The diversity, the need for experiences, bringing other things into it. And experiencing other people's scenarios too. A lot of it is roughly the same. I remember playing with a group of friends around ten years of age and we played lots of games that contained a very mild flavour of what I do now. There were three of us and my friend's father was the headmaster of the school. After school *finished we had it as our playground. We'd play control games. He had a little sister, two years younger, who was very bossy and powerful for her age. I look back and see how that could be a possible source for my interests.*

'*It was seventy pounds for an hour-long session back when I was first getting involved. A lot of money. My sessions weren't that frequent but once I found the person who I thought was very good, very experienced (now there are so many the quality isn't really there) I went more often. Years ago it took something to find someone who knew what they were doing. Someone who had a deeper feeling for it. I was lucky to find somebody who became close to me. She's retired now but we're still close. Through her I got more involved in the scene. It was a beautiful experience for me because I'd come to London and found myself with all these people who felt the same as me and it was nothing to be lonely about, or ashamed of. It was accepted among these people and that was good enough. I had a freedom suddenly. That experience helped me take it to extremes, no inhibitions.*

'*Now I see myself as a fairly hard player. I pick and choose what it is I want to play at but within those boundaries I like to stretch myself. It's not just about pain, it's about the psychology of it too, and perhaps that's the most important thing. A mistress might shackle you and then say "I'm going to keep you here for ever." And it begins to play with your mind. You think, "Is she serious?" Unless you know somebody very well, then maybe they are serious. If you go to somebody who doesn't inspire that fear in you then it isn't going to work.*'

Some slaves are married, or in relationships, so they have to keep visits to me a secret. I can't mark them in any way. One ingenious way of getting around this is if they wear wet shorts; this prevents any marking. Some men can be in a happy relationship but they come to me to talk, to get things off their chest, discuss things that they can't discuss with their wives.

They need something different. Searching for that extra bit of the puzzle that they can't get at home.

One guy called Henry wears just pants and I'll wear a leather cat suit and a hood and he just wants to cuddle me while I'm in that outfit. It's quite a learning curve when you think about all the things they like. It's mind-boggling, the perv permutations that exist. They all want me to piss on them, that's the strange thing. They like it. I don't know why. I suppose it's because they get a glimpse of you, Mistress's divine parts, which is I suppose understandable.

I had this problem with a former partner I used to dominate in session. Sometimes you have to detach the relationship from this special world of servitude you've created. I commanded Benson once to untie a rope from a bench.

He said, 'I can't do it, darling.'

Immediately I slapped him across the face and said, 'I'm not your darling, I'm your Mistress. Now do it!'

And he said, 'I can't do it.'

I grabbed him by the throat and said, 'If we were in a proper session you wouldn't be allowed to talk to me like that. Get your head in the right place or I'm stopping now.'

I left him for five minutes and when I returned he was on his hands and knees in the kowtow position, arms outstretched, head on the floor. A traditional, submissive, *I fucked up* position. He was okay after that. It's very difficult to step outside of a relationship but it's important if you are to stay true to the codes of BDSM and not dilute the power you possess in session. It's interesting how some slaves can't switch off and give themselves to the moment. After all, one of the main reasons for putting yourself in that position is to give up all control to somebody else.

Slaves can apply to be Body Slaves but it's not usually something I permit. I'll usually wait until a slave has come to me for six sessions – to demonstrate a willingness to be faithful to me as their sole mistress, to display a real commitment to be servile – before I consider allowing them to give me physical worship. I might tell them, no, I've changed my mind, wait until the next session. Or body worship might involve my ankle or my hand. They're parts of my body – get on with it. If he's disappointed by that, then he's not a true slave. A true slave will understand that he gets nothing unless I decide to give it, and he should be grateful for whatever is thrown his way. If they're dedicated, they'll do it. These are my rules.

Body Slaves are also known as Toys, or Boys. Lots of mistresses have favourites that they grant sexual favours to, but mistresses don't always sleep with their slaves. They may allow sexual favours, perhaps allow intimate contact, as in bottom worship or pussy worship, so that Mistress is getting pleasure. But that's only if they're into the sensual, physical side of things – it's important to understand that not all clients are – you have to remember that it's not necessarily a scene that is directly involved with sex, which is where people outside of BDSM show their ignorance. It's just as much, if not more, about punishment and discipline and control for a lot of slaves. They aren't really interested in any sexual involvement. Choosing a Body Slave is like choosing a boyfriend in many ways. You have to be drawn to them.

When they serve me in public, at a fetish club for example, they must not talk to any other women without first seeking my permission. Sometimes I might insist that they deliver a written request to me. A mistress can do what she likes. She can have any slave for any number of tasks, chores or any type of servitude.

I think that some slaves resist the temptation to offer themselves for body worship because they fear they might lose interest in me, because suddenly I'm no longer this aloof unattainable Goddess. I need to be something they cannot have in order to increase their tension and maintain that magical mysterious separation. I'm not like any other woman. I know that for sure. The sexual fantasies I create for them are intense. I'm their whore and lover, mistress and wife figure. Polite and lady-like most of the time, but I can kill them slowly with my words. As one said to me, 'You're a lady on my arm and a whore in my bed.' There are no limits for me; I will do anything sexually that most wives would not dream of. This is my greatest love, to tease them. Some would say it's sluttish, but I know that's not true. Men have had erections simply by watching me put on my leather opera gloves.

I'm very in tune with my body and a slight tickle of my neck can set off four or five hours of passion. I'd like to think that I'm dangerous but great fun with it. I love dangerous games. I will explore anything, even strangulation; one of my ex-boyfriends would sometimes fuck me while we simulated hanging.

From Slave Benson's diary:

Woke up feeling very aroused but had to get up to attend meetings in the City. Permanently semi-firm all day. Mistress's exercises have certainly got the blood flowing again.

Sexual frustration led to me not paying attention in meetings. Finally managed to get home and before tea laid on my bed, twisting my aching nipples with my left hand, remembering Mistress's body and the pleasure she took from me. The way she was dressed, head to foot in black leather, urging me to satisfy her. I lay before her, at her mercy, as she played with, teased and tormented me. I imagine her as commander of a castle, with all of her slave boys chained up, suspended from a hanging bar. She takes me using her double-headed dildo. Real experiences and fantasies merge in my mind. I do not come, as I have been ordered to save my milk for her later, and my mind wonders what her dungeon will look like, and what she might be wearing.

Punishments:
Failing to replenish Mistress' wine glass – Nipple clamps
Forgetting to buy Mistress flowers – Boot licking
Being cheeky – Face slap
Talking about another mistress – 50 x cane

Looking at a woman in a sluttish outfit – 20 x paddle and airing cupboard for half an hour
Rubbing Mistress' stockings without permission – Cock and ball torture

Benson homework:
The letter sent to me explained clearly that I was to call a mobile phone at precisely 19.30 hours on Friday. I gave the password.

'Applicant, please answer this question.' There was a pause. The instructions had said I was to remain silent. After a short pause the voice continued.

'Do you wish to enter Camp X-ray?'

'I do.'

'Code word?'

'Spider,' I answered.

'You wish to make an application and agree to the tribute?' she continued.

'I do.'

I was given further instructions and details of what would happen.

Three days later I found myself waiting at the appointed rendezvous. I looked around nervously. The park was totally empty, but then I saw a woman sitting on a park bench. As I approached she stood and walked towards me. She was dressed head to foot in black leather.

'Good evening, Benson,' she said.

I nodded. 'Commandant.'

She slid her arm through mine and I felt something hard and metallic jab into my ribs. Glancing down I noticed a pistol nestled into my ribs.

'Walk with me,' she said and we marched towards a block of flats. During the walk she checked all the details given to me. Soon we arrived at a front door, which opened. As we entered, a blue nylon bag was put over my head and the drawstring tightened. Her gloved hands guided me forwards.

'Strip,' she commanded.

I heard some rustling sounds, then the sound of something sticky being readied.

A cold baton touched my shoulder.

'Welcome to Camp X-ray. I am sure we are in for a very interesting time. Kneel.'

Releasing the drawstring she pulled up the hood far enough to reveal my lips. Her black leather gloved hands smoothed three pieces of elasticated plaster over my mouth. Taking me by the elbow, she guided me on to a latex-covered bed. It was only when my legs banged into some metal bars I realised I was in a cell. Her hands touched my skin as the commandant bound me hand and foot. Finally a pair of headphones were placed over my ears. Strange music flooded them. I felt someone come close and a leather-clad hand clamped something across my mouth and nose, soaked in a pungent chemical which had me spinning out of control . . .

The second time a client comes to see me, they have to bring a book with their slave name written on the first page and they'll use this to put down their fantasies. I'll add punishments or mark their work, like a very unusual teacher. For example, I'll write that they must tie their balls up for four hours and write about my first visit to their home. As far as I know, no other mistress does this. It comes from the experiments I did with Graham at the Silk Planet.

From Slave Benson's book:

Manacled to the wall, Mistress lets fly with her quirt. She assures me I am about to suffer. Six hundred and one blows later I lie at her booted feet, begging for mercy. I bottle it, because I am beginning to enjoy agony and a sexual release previously unsurpassed. She promises me I will be rewarded. Her vanilla mixed with the leather of my hood tastes warm and moist. Sucking on my gag, my eyes obscured, manacled, I am left to contemplate my fate.

The way I came up with this idea was connected to value for money. A session with me costs £150 and if you're not very wealthy, once a month can be quite a struggle. When I had my own dungeon, at my place in Bromley, people would come along with their tribute and I'd keep them there for two or three hours as opposed to the usual one hour. Because I like what I do. I'll do it for nothing, and I have done. I was wondering about what I could do to keep them interested, to keep them thinking about me even when a session was over. Because if they're thinking of me, at some point they'll book another session. I want them to be excited, curious, on their toes all the time. So if they write in the book they must be thinking of you, and the sessions they've had, or the sessions that are yet to come. While they're watching TV with their wives and children they're thinking about what they have to write in the book. On top of that I'll insist that they report in. So everybody is given a specific date and time when they must contact me in some way. They have to text or email me once a week, phone in once a week – so they're in contact with me one way or another. In this way I'm on their minds all the time.

Sometimes I'd be making love to my partner and I'd call one of the slaves, maybe three in the morning, and they'd have to listen to me being fucked. I'd usually get a text back saying 'Mistress that was fantastic. Thank you for the late night call.'

I like playing little tricks like that. I might send someone a text at one in the morning instructing them to bark like a dog for ten minutes, or wear their collar and hood, or put pegs on their nipples. Someone like Slave Daphne – a total slave who is currently undergoing feminisation training with me – will always do as I say.

This is a marriage ceremony uniting Daphne to the Web of Princess Spider.

Do you Daphne, now in lifelong chastity, promise to love, honour, worship and obey Princess Spider and the Web, forsaking all others for as long as you shall live?

I do, Mistress
Daphne, in becoming the bride of the Web, do you
totally renounce your previous male identity and
complete your transformation into womanhood?
I do, Mistress
As a bride, Daphne, do you promise to faithfully serve
the Web for the remainder of your days?
I do, Mistress
Repeat after me:
*I Daphne, as the Bride of the Web, promise to faithfully
serve the Web in its entirety without a thought to my
own needs for the rest of my days.*

From The Birth of Slave Daphne:

It all began some thirty years ago when my life was turned upside
down. At the time, and for reasons unknown to me, I was
compelled to visit a mistress and be dominated by her. This was
something so foreign to me at the time but the urge got stronger
as the days went by. Eventually I located a mistress, which was not
easy in those days, made an appointment and visited her. After a
short chat I soon found myself undressed, with my backside
receiving a caning. To my surprise I felt such great joy and a great
sense of release as this happened.

I found myself seeking other mistresses. As I did so I found
myself becoming even more subservient and I realised that what I
was doing was acknowledging the superiority of women over
men.

Over the years, the mistresses came and went and I was
introduced to further treatment such as whips and torture to my
nipples and genitals. This was becoming my way of life. I did make
the odd mistake, such as saying that I was able to take more
punishment than I actually could. Do this and you will soon learn
otherwise. I did find that some mistresses were good and some of
these I visited more than once. There were those that were
moderate and those that were downright awful.

There are those out there who are true sadists but do not advertise as such and on more than one occasion I found myself in a threatening situation. The major problem was that for many years the clubs were not open to single men and so there was nobody I could talk to. It was a lonely path to walk. I tried to be more selective in my choice of mistress and tried to explain my need more explicitly when talking to them on the phone. In this, showing respect can count for a lot.

Then 18 months ago I met Princess Spider. On our first meeting I instinctively knew I had found perfection. We quickly discovered that we both like to play hard and there were so many more compatible things between us. A rigid slave contract was quickly drawn up, a contract that gives my Princess total ownership of me that I signed with such great joy because it meant we could begin our great voyage of discovery. Whatever limits there were before when I played were now non-existent.

When I signed the contract I was given the slave name Daphne but didn't realise why. It eventually became clear. At the beginning, my Princess had recognised an extremely strong feminine side to me and was now proceeding to feminise me. Out went my old male way of life. In came the pretty clothes and the make-up. I am now only known as Daphne, my old male name having been discarded.

I have also been locked into full-time chastity because what I have between my legs is totally redundant. I truly am a feminine slave to my Princess and I am proud of it. It was difficult and lonely being on my own but that is in the past. I am now content and at peace. I have found the perfection I sought and I have found it in my mistress, Princess Spider.

Slave Daphne

The way I treat a slave might have a link to his background. I like to find out about a slave's upbringing and interests. It might not seem important, but sometimes you can unlock a fetish or a desire through those elements that other people might not have tried. It can be quite an interesting seam to mine. They might not even be aware of that facet of their personality. I like unlocking doors. I like to open people up to opportunities they didn't believe existed.

I met the slave I called Benson when he was married. He craved hard sessions but couldn't partake in them because he couldn't be marked. He was with me and another mistress. We'd doubled up in this particular session. I understood he was from a military background so I decided to give him a harsh ritualistic interrogation. I tied his hands roughly behind him and taped a bin liner over his back and filled it with ice water. I made him kiss knives, I put guns in his mouth, I really brutalised him. When he turned over, all of the iced water drenched him. There was a lot of tension. He said it was the best session he'd ever had. The other mistress had been quite nervous about being so extreme with him and said she'd never dominated anybody like that before.

'But he's an ex-soldier,' I said. 'He can take it.'

Benson is one example of a slave who can push his way to the head of my list. I'm not an ice queen. I do fall in love, and if I'm attracted to a slave, I don't see anything wrong with that. There was something about him. I thought he was really nice. I saw him again on a hotel visit. He wanted a kidnap scene. So I put tape on his mouth, and tied him up. I like peculiarities, it helps to disarm the slaves and mess with their heads, so I made him wear a yellow stocking on one leg and a pink stocking on the other. I sat and watched him, tied him on the bed and left him and thought, yeah, I'm going to have him. I went to the bathroom, stripped off down to underwear, black lacy bra and knickers. Stockings. I went back into the room, straddled him – he was getting aroused by now – and tore off the tape from his lips. I kissed him and I thought, I'll know by how he returns this whether he wants me too. And he gave me a full-on sexy kiss. So I said, 'Mistress has decided that pleasure is going to be reversed tonight. Instead of yours, it's going to be mine.' And I took him. It was amazing.

I had tried to show him I liked him earlier, because we went for dinner first, and I held his hand. I was granting him access to an intimacy that few have been allowed.

Later, he said, 'Mistresses never hold hands with their slaves. I knew something funny was going on.'

The slave is in a strange position. He (or she) has to shrug off their everyday skin for an hour or two, and become something that is utterly alien to their perceived selves. The mistress is who she is, who she wants to be. The slave has to get into role very quickly in order to succeed at what he's doing, and to enjoy it. You have to leave your everyday existence behind. You are entering a brand new world for a little while. Nothing from your old world should follow you inside. It's that step from the mundane to the bizarre that separates us. At four o'clock you might be on the phone tying up a deal or chairing a meeting in an office. At five o'clock you might be in the dungeon having hot wax poured down the crack of your arse. It's difficult to do but in order to immerse yourself fully, to prepare yourself and allow yourself to know the beauty of submission, you have to assume that slave mentality.

PERMISSION TO SPEAK: Slave Rooster

Rooster has always been my straight guy. We run a company, Spifilms, together, so it's not a conventional Mistress/Slave relationship. He's not a typical slave ... actually he's a bad slave. He never does as he's told. But when I get depressed he can pull me out of it.

'We met a couple of years ago while I was working on a television series in which she performed – I'm a director of television films. At the time I didn't notice anything but she apparently took an interest in me. We didn't meet again for a couple of months after that until I became involved in this TV series about fetishes and knew nothing about it, I'd inherited it from another director, so it wasn't my subject. But I did some

research and the film was made and it was successful and Princess took part in some of the episodes. It wasn't until the middle of the year, after a succession of emails, that I jokingly said, "I really should experience this."

'We literally, formally, went through all the motions. So I booked the appointment and thought I knew what to expect and away from my own territory I was quite apprehensive. I knew her well enough to know that she wasn't going to hurt me or anything like that. When I turned up for this session, it didn't transpire quite as I had imagined at all. I was seduced. I thought I'd just come for a session. I was very nervous and didn't realise that she wanted me. It wasn't a normal session. I resisted it a few times, because I was married. We became lovers.

'The relationship and the work thing came together which made it quite powerful. We set about trying to do certain things. We came up with the idea for the TV series that became Dominatrix Reloaded.

'I've always had a great belief in her ability, not only as a dominatrix but also in terms of someone with spontaneity. She has a very fertile imagination. When we were filming it was extraordinary, we were coming up with ideas all the time. We'd work hard during the day but had a ball at the same time. I was seeing her as a mistress, and a lover, and a business partner, a quite extraordinary combination.

'My sessions with her weren't so formal. At the time I didn't really need to make an appointment, because I was living with her. The attraction was that she'd grab me by the neck and order me downstairs. You knew what she wanted. She'd say strip. Or force you to your knees. And she'd beat you but she always knew what I liked or what I didn't like.

'I've always been involved with powerful women. But in slave mode, it's more formal than with someone not involved businesswise, as I am with Princess Spider. The demarcation is more blurred.

'We see each other a lot so most sessions are an extension

of the working day. In the past I've escorted her to various parties and clubs and often she's needed someone to help with her demonstrations. On one occasion we were filming in the south of France and I was talking to a slave who was acting in the film. He was interested in the quirt but had never experienced it. He wanted me to ask Spider if she would use it on him. When he saw Spider attacking my back with it at a demonstration later he held up his hands and said: "No way." The thing about the quirt is that it looks worse than it is.

'I prefer erotic play. Whether she derives some form of power exchange from it I don't know. What I do know is that she has never put me through anything I didn't like. It's a much softer experience for me because it's less formal.

'With regards to the whole fetish scene, I can take it or leave it. I find it mildly interesting in terms of the people. There are a lot of great characters. And visually it is a fascinating experience. In session I'll let go and for one hour I'll enter the world and be a part of it. But if you took it away from me tomorrow I wouldn't miss it.

'This informs the way she plays with me. As soon as I get into the dungeon she takes my sight away from me and puts me in a state of confusion. She uses my awareness against me and she'll tease me a lot. One moment she'll be whispering something in my ear and the next she's talking to me from the other side of the room. Dialogue is very important. She's always talking to you, laying traps for you. She has this soft voice and a harsh voice and an evil laugh. It's amazing to hear her flit around this vocal range. I don't think she's even working at this, or conceiving a plan of action. I think it's all natural to her. She's good at building the intensity, like someone writing a story. She knows how to structure a session. She's very playful, very good at doing what she does when she's in her domain. The sessions aren't so much about me as her. I take a great deal of pleasure, when I'm not in a blindfold, from watching her reaction to doing things. She might be sticking *needles in me, for example, and I will watch her face, because she's so absorbed by the moment it's fascinating to see. It's a kind of caring, curious expression, quite unusual. She's investing her whole being in whatever activity she's involved with.*

'*She loves men a lot. That might sound funny when you consider how brutal she can be with them, but it's true. She respects them. She's not like a lot of dommes who treat men like shit. She'll be firm with men, but she gives them the benefit of the doubt.*

'*Reciprocity is very important to her. She wants the sessions to be as much about her enjoyment as her slaves'. It's important for her to immerse herself in the things she's doing because that means that the experience for the slaves is going to be that much more intense. She's not in it for the money. She lives it. She's absorbed by it.*'

Beyond the Body Slaves is an elite bunch of men who are my Praetorian Guard. My special circle. These are five slaves who have a special relationship with me. My lover is one, my ex-lover another. The other three are slaves who have proved themselves to be utterly submissive, dedicated to me and my world, and willing to go to extraordinary measures to serve me, at any time of the day or night, 365 days of the year. They are prepared to put their own lives on hold, or even turn their backs on their lives in order to please me. One slave left his wife of fourteen years for me. I don't condone this kind of extreme behaviour, but that kind of devotion is what I need in order to allow someone in to my inner sanctum. They each have to build their own altar of respect.

Twin has a little Buddha figure with a ceremonial knife and when we play at his flat we have incense burning there. Daphne has a huge shrine because he lives alone. He has images of me all over the wall. He's really gone over the top. It's fantastic.

PERMISSION TO SPEAK: Slave Rooster

'Before I met Princess Spider I knew this world existed and roughly what it represented. But if you'd said to me a month before "Would I take the quirt, and enjoy it?" I'd have thought you were mad. The only difference is that I have never served another mistress and I would never serve another mistress. If I never see Princess Spider again I would never do it again. I think from that point of view that's what makes me, in the capacity of Slave Rooster, a very bad slave but also a very devoted slave.

'It is very difficult. Really it's a terrible mix-up. I loved her, still love her, and I'm devoted to her. I personally don't see quite the boundary as perhaps she does. The difference is that as a slave in a session the devotion is such that I trust her completely. Without question, with the quirt, she can kill you. She is a very powerful, physical person. Mentally, too, she has the ability to utterly confuse you, even someone like me who I believe to be quite logical and organised, she can have me tied up in metaphorical knots. It's a complete trust thing and I don't personally believe I would enjoy it as much if it wasn't her.

'We've had a roaring old 18 months and it's been full throttle in a lot of things. I would like to think – as she does – that businesswise we have a strong bond. In my 53 years I can't think of anyone I've shared so much with in such a short space of time. I left my wife of fourteen years for this woman. I love my wife, and still see her, but it's been a big upheaval. The decision to leave her was the biggest I've ever faced. But my feeling was such that I did it.'

An introductory letter from a slave:

Dear Princess Spider

I am into bondage, helplessness, physical abuse, but not verbal abuse/humiliation.

I like the idea of coming into your web and being captured by being overpowered (kicked, slapped, punched, lassoed), forcibly stripped and trussed up.

I might be interrogated, maybe to find out what I did in the Army. I'm afraid I can't remember my number, but I do remember my rank.

I am not good with weights on balls or straightforward corporal punishment on my bum, but being whipped on my belly and chest you may enjoy. I am afraid that any marks that don't disappear by the next day would be embarrassing for me.

I expect I would be buggered, maybe singed with a cigarette. My nipples, I feel sure, would come in for some attention.

I like 'good guy, bad guy' and respond well to care and sweet words after pain and suffering. I talk a lot so a gag would be needed some of the time. Speech deprivation and breath control may be some of the things you employ.

Above all I like to be tied up in different positions. I am sure you have things you like doing best, so please indulge and enjoy yourself.

Slave John

I'm always smiling when I'm in the middle of a session. I treat it professionally, but it's also great fun for me. Because I do it so much as a part of my normal life. Sometimes you can feel randy after a session, depending on who it is, other times your mind is just blown away. Normally, in a session, I feel quite drained. It's tough work. I listen to their hearts, offer care throughout it, keep an eye on them at the same time as beat the living daylights out of them. I'll do three sessions and then go off to sleep for three hours. It's a mentally and physically demanding activity.

Every time I see Twin, we play. Either me dommeing him or him dommeing me. It's like a drug. You want more and more and more. Sometimes we have vanilla sex but I'll put him in a scissor lock, throw him over on his back, pinch his nipples and say, 'Right, little boy . . .' and he'll say: 'Oh my God, we're off again.' But Twin is a creative guy and he helps me explore more about myself through the games we play. It's so exciting, and I like adventures.

Twin, after a session, finds it almost like a workout. He feels energised, euphoric, and it's the same for me too. It's almost as if I don't want to stop. Sometimes we'll have sessions at home that last all night till six in the morning. We just want to experiment with pain levels and play in as many directions as we can take it. He tests my levels too, but he's still frightened of really hurting me. But I tell him he can be as brutal as he likes. I've played hard for many years now and I can take a lot. What he does to me half the time is no more than tickle me. If you're going to hit me with something, hit me.

It's like ten orgasms at once when our sessions hit that zone where everything feels fresh and right and true. Twin is in a daze sometimes. We have a small area to play in at his place, and sometimes being in a confined space is better, because you're more controlled. You have to be more inventive. Our best sessions have occurred during these times, far away from a well-kitted atmospheric dungeon.

PERMISSION TO SPEAK: Slave Twin

'We met at a party. I was helping the mistress who was organising the party. I was designing the artwork for an advert for her and she had sent me all these images of the mistresses who were going to be involved. And one of them was Princess Spider. Immediately I saw her I thought she was nice. I was attracted to her straight away but I didn't think too much about it. It's a big leap from becoming acquainted with a mistress to getting to know her on a different level, so it didn't really enter the equation at that point. I didn't want to cross those lines of etiquette. They probably get it all the time. I don't want to be just another hustler.

'When the party started there were about six mistresses there and I'd checked Princess Spider out when she arrived and thought she looked a bit severe. I thought, I hope she doesn't get hold of me tonight because I'll be in trouble. I saw her walk through and the first thing I heard her say was: "Where's my strap-on?" And I thought, Oh my God, I've got to stay away from her.

'I was playing elsewhere and I went off to the bathroom and suddenly I was whisked into the room where she was, put on the bench and things started to happen. I glanced at her and she looked amazing. There's something about her, something sensuous and I was attracted deeply to it. I think she liked me too because we were pretty inseparable for the rest of the party.

'When I left I had her telephone number but I wasn't sure if it was something I should pursue. I was attracted to her as a person first, not as a mistress. And that was how I wanted to see her. I wasn't really aware of her status within the scene because I wasn't really a part of it.

'When we met again I wasn't sure if she was that interested. I wanted to serenade her. So I went to her, having booked a session. I had that as my back-up in case my serenading plan failed. I bought her perfume and flowers and arrived feeling nervous. Our texting had been getting hot, the hints were all there. So we had a bit of a session and I took her out for dinner.

'She had her entourage and we all went out as a group later and by then I began to know a little bit about who she was. I wasn't aware of how much of a public image she had. But I could see she had something quite special. I also knew she had a reputation for being severe, and that was both good and bad, because I didn't know how severe I wanted to go, even though I had been looking out for someone who could take me to the next level. I needed someone who was capable of controlling me. Outside of that she's incredibly sensuous and able to play with your mind. She looks for triggers all the time. You'll be having a conversation and she'll be taking mental notes to see what would work with you in a session. She'll watch how your eyes or your body react. It's a little interrogation technique. She's been to where submissives go to so she knows it well.

'She's one of the best I've ever met. Some of the concepts she

*has, like the homework books, are great things. Because even
though you are no longer with her, you're still under her
control. She's one crazy woman. But she's also very sensitive
and caring too. She's the most sexual woman I've ever met. She
has a great appetite. It's hard work …'*

With a partner, BDSM is great because it's a fascinating
extension of sex. It can be very erotic. The other night with
Twin I was in white mules, which is not really me but he likes
me in them, and a black nightie. He had his cock and balls tied
up in leather twine and I'd put a leash on him and I was
making him do things while I had hold of the leash. I told him
to masturbate and he was trying to and I gave him
encouragement by sticking my foot in his mouth, so he was
licking my toes and I asked him do you want to see something
better, so I stood over him so he could see up my nightie. And
I'm saying to him, 'I want you to come for me, I like to watch.'
Torments like that are intense and exciting – in the end I had
to put my feet on his cock in order to make him come because
he's a foot worshipper – he was so into it he was perspiring. I
can see by looking at his eyes what he likes. Afterwards he
said, 'My God, you did all my favourite things.' It's not rocket
science. It's just reading the person you're with.

Clients are the lifeblood of a mistress's existence. But they
don't half piss you around sometimes. I get a lot of
unreasonable requests from some of them, especially the first-
timers. Mainly to do with sex.

What slaves do, and I always get this whether it's telephone,
text, email, any communication, they say: *Mistress I want this,
I can take this, I want to do that.*

A guy called Michael got in touch with me and said he
wanted to be pierced all over with needles, but mainly his face.
He wanted to drink in session which I am not keen on and will
not allow unless I know the person and I am confident he can
take it. I agreed that he could have one drink of vodka –

although he'd obviously been drinking before he came to see me. So he came into the dungeon, and I put him in a collar and cuffs and got him down on his knees.

Realising that I was going to have to mark him facially, I loosened his collar and put him in a sling that was hanging from the ceiling. He had sent these emails to me going on and on about this fantastic fantasy he had about being punctured in the face by lots of needles, but I just had a feeling he wouldn't go through with it. At least he was paying more than the usual tribute for this unusual session, so I had to give him his due. I had purchased about 200 needles – three-inch hypodermic needles – some surgical spirit and plenty of sanitary wipes because you never know how much blood is going to be shed. I put a surgical mask over his face and tried to help him to get relaxed.

So I started gently playing with him, pinching his nipples, lightly flogging him just to get him distracted, and he said, impatiently: 'Mistress, could you do this thing with the needles now?'

And I said: 'I'm in charge. I've got the brief. I know what you want. But you have to relax first. I need you to get your head in the right place.'

I could see by the way he was holding onto the straps that he was still quite tense. After a while, though, he had loosened up a little so I felt it was safe to insert the first needle in his face, just near his eyebrow. I put two more in, all of them close together, and suddenly he couldn't handle any more. He had paid for a two-hour session and was there for little more than an hour. It was annoying in a way because I just couldn't understand why he'd tried to go for more than he was capable of. He clearly had no grasp of his own pain threshold. It was quite obvious to me that he would wimp out. I'm actually glad he did, because I wasn't comfortable about doing it, and I would refuse to do anything like that again. But you have to build up to these extreme levels. I've had boys who couldn't take the cane, and others who can take 500 straight off. For

Michael it was just a fantasy, and should have stayed a fantasy. It was a weird thing to want to do.

Another slave called Ray called and asked if I could knock him out. I said, 'Yes, give me a baseball bat and I'll quite happily knock you out.'

But of course he didn't mean that. He wanted me to get a tourniquet and strangle him. I had to tie the tourniquet – which was this length of rubber hose – and then put a bag over his head containing a cotton wool ball soaked in amyl nitrate. I said we'd do a test, to see what happened, so I did it and his face went red, then blue, and he was almost out so I let go of the hose. So I knew what was going to happen. I coaxed him back, massaging him gently, and I listened to his heartbeat. It was going a bit faster than usual so I decided to leave it a bit before I did it again. I got him talking to me and I said, 'When you go I'm going to tap you on your face. If you don't respond I'll slap you. And if you die today, I know how to get rid of a body so don't give me any shit.'

I was really terrified because it was the first time I'd done any kind of multiple knock-out scenario. I'd knocked boys out before, but not continually. When I was tying the tourniquet, the fear went away. I was getting a kick out of it. The risk was minimal, but it was there. A human life was in my hands; he was depending on me to revive him at the crucial moment. I was suddenly enjoying it; I know I could have killed this guy if he wasn't healthy – he was a bodybuilder and a bouncer so he was in pretty good shape. I did it about four times and thought, that's it – I've had enough. So I told him I needed a rest. 'I want to be honest, I've never done this before,' I told him. 'I need some time to think about what has happened here.'

And I never saw him again because I thought it was too much to risk. It was a nice experience, in hindsight. It was interesting to see how the body behaves when you're rendered unconscious. It was quite a power kick to do this to a big strong man. He was saying he could go on and on, and I said to him, 'Yes, I know *you* can, but *I can't*.' I had to draw the line in that situation. Don't try this at home ...

The annoying callers who just request sex do it because they're not well educated. They don't really know what a dominatrix does. They can download lots of stories about me from the internet where they read about how I've had Body Slaves give me pussy worship, bottom worship, thigh worship, breast worship. They think that when they're alone with me in session that's a normal part of proceedings. But what they don't realise is that what happens in a club, when Mistress is having a good time, is not like a private session. Sex doesn't come into it. And when it does, a lot of the time sex can be used as just another form of punishment or domination.

From Slave Daphne's diary:

Saturday
I wasn't sure what to expect this evening. I knew that I was going to wear my new skirt for the first time and I was thrilled about that. My Princess had told me beforehand that I would be sucking a lot of cock and to my surprise I felt quite excited about this. I couldn't help wondering if there was another side to me that was waiting to be released and because of the thoughts I was having, would it be tonight when it happened?

I met my Princess at East Croydon and we were soon at the venue. I was introduced to the other mistresses and made to feel welcome. Although I didn't know what was in store for me I felt totally relaxed but then I always do when in the presence of my Princess. Very soon the command was given to get changed. I felt so comfortable as I put on my hold-ups and skirt. Finally, wrist and ankle cuffs and the slave collar went on.

After meeting the other slaves and displaying my backside so that they could see the effects of punishment given by my Princess there was a briefing on what we could and could not do. We were then split up among the mistresses and I was so glad that my Princess made sure I was with her and Mistress Alicia because of what followed.

I was introduced to the strap-ons by having to suck them, taking them deep into my mouth. I was then commanded to suck the other slave's cock. Somehow this seemed to be such a natural things to do and I enjoyed taking that cock in my mouth. Then my Princess said what are now, to me, magic words: 'I'm going to fuck Daphne.'

As I lay on the bench I felt my hole being lubricated and then felt my Princess enter me. I realised this was what I had secretly longed for as my Princess pushed the strap-on deep inside and began to fuck me. As my Princess slid in deeper I was taken totally out of my mind. It was such a beautiful moment.

After some time my Princess finished fucking me and left me in the hands of Mistress Alicia. I was instantly ordered to carry on sucking cock and as I did so she started to use a dildo on me which I later discovered was about 9" long and I was told that every inch of it went inside. As I was being fucked I was not only sucking cock but sucking it greedily.

Eventually the fucking stopped. Mistress Alicia produced another dildo and in front of my eyes started to slide it into her pussy. After a while I was instructed to lick the dildo clean. By now I felt that I had died and gone to heaven. The fucking may have stopped (much to my disappointment) but the sucking hadn't. For around the next two hours there was hardly a moment when I didn't have a cock in my mouth and I sucked deeply until my jaws ached. I found myself wanting a cock to explode and release its milk into my mouth but unfortunately this didn't happen.

We had a break for a while to chill out. That is, the mistresses had a break while the slaves carried on sucking and licking. Then it was back upstairs for more sucking and being sucked. There was one memorable moment when one of the slaves was sucking me and I had a wonderful view of my Princess fucking Mistress Alicia. It was sheer perfection. It was wonderful to see my Princess so happy. I was full of joy.

The evening was drawing to an end all too quickly and I started to panic. I found myself begging my Princess for her to fuck me and much to my great relief she said she would. I cannot describe

PRINCESS SPIDER: TRUE EXPERIENCES OF A DOMINATRIX

the immense pleasure and contentment that I felt as she entered me and went deep inside with every stroke. I truly did not want that moment to end. Sadly it did but my feelings were so intense at that time.

However the evening was not quite over as my Princess decided to use her quirt on me. With all that had been going on, and now this, I was truly in heaven and I had such beautiful feelings running through me. After a while Mistress Wolf joined in but did not have the finesse that my Princess had. The number of strokes had reached 76 when it was all over. The time had come to wrap up the party. It was time to get dressed and return home, which I did on such an incredible high.

In addition to being a total pain slave to my Princess something else had happened during the evening. My Princess had set free the feminine side that was within me. This was a side I was not aware of but I suspect that my Princess was and had decided to bring it out. I felt so happy about this turn of events and now truly appreciate the slave name of Daphne.

My Princess has said that it would be a good idea for me to wear feminine underwear full time. I have wonderful thoughts about going shopping, my Princess helping me to select girly clothing not just for daytime but maybe at night when I am in bed. Having to try on clothing in the shop would truly be public humiliation, especially if the assistants knew that the clothing was intended for me.

That release of my feminine side, coupled with all that had happened, brought something else out. It has shown just how total a slut I am. The slut who, in addition to being caned, whipped and tortured, also wants to be fucked severely with strap-ons, dildos and cocks and wants to suck cocks until climax.

There is a postscript to the evening. The following day my Princess received an email from a mistress criticising the tone of the evening set by my Princess and Mistress Alicia. From what I saw and heard there were no complaints from any of the slaves during the evening. In fact, without exception, they were all highly delighted. Had my Princess and Mistress Alicia not been there, the whole evening would have been very low-key and there would have been many glum faces. It seemed to me that among the other mistresses, inexperience was very high on the list.

There's also the slight possibility of danger. When I had my dungeon in South London, a great place, it was above a fetish shop – the shop is still there – I was conducting a session with Slave Mouse and Slave Benson, a dressing-up day when Benson was a referee and Mouse was dressed as a girl in a nice red PVC outfit with a hood.

Mouse was on the medical chair and Benson was strapped up in a harness. And this guy just walked in. I didn't notice at first but he had his cock out and he was rubbing it. He said: 'Mistress, I'd really like a session.'

I said, 'One, put that away. Two, you don't interrupt my sessions up here or come in here without an appointment. Who let you in?'

He said it was the lady downstairs looking after the shop.

I said, 'Well you're not allowed to be here now. Get out – this is not about sexual services. These people are paying for my time and you're interrupting.' I said it a bit nastier than that, actually, but I released the boys and went downstairs to sort it out with the woman running the shop. There's no locking door to the dungeon, that was one problem. I saw the guy walk straight out of the shop and the woman had never sent him up. There was just a connecting door and he let himself in. It could have been quite nasty.

On a lighter note, I get annoyed when people don't stay in the position they're supposed to when I'm punishing them. Some people wriggle about when they're being caned which can cause the cane to connect with their back instead of their bottom, and that can be dangerous, especially if you catch them around the kidneys.

Meeting a client for the first time can be a very nerve-racking affair. The first thing I do when I know a new boy is on the way? Smoke like a trooper! I'm usually quite nervous. At the dungeon I take between 10–15 minutes and wipe down all the surfaces that might be touched by a human body. Especially the whips, because if they're not clean and you've cut someone with it in a previous session, you don't know what you might be passing on. I would have already received a letter or text from them, explaining their preferences, so I'll put on some music suitable to their fetish, a couple of hours before they were coming, so that I could get into the mood. The music depends on the fetish they describe. If it's caning, you'll put something upbeat on; if they like foot worship, something softer, calmer. If it's a newcomer, you'll have a selection of CDs because the chances are they will want to try everything.

If they want me in leather I'll go through my leather collection and choose the most comfortable outfit for the day depending on how I am feeling. I've had requests for a leather catsuit when it's been 90 degrees in the shade. It's hellish. Sometimes I have candles lit, sometimes not. It's different strokes for different folks, no pun intended.

Some go straight to the dungeon, some I talk to first. In the past when I've had more flexible time I would talk to them in their street clothes and then send them off to get dressed, then talk to them again in the dungeon about their confessions, and find out if they were happy with what was about to happen to them. I'd get them to write down anything they didn't want to try, what they were allergic to, any particular concerns or worries. It's kind of like vetting them. From what they say or write I can tell whether I'll have them as a named slave or a normal slave. It depends how dedicated and polite they are.

I try to use the room like a clock, or a figure of eight. I rotate, keep things interesting, keep moving them around, putting them in the stocks, the cage, on the floor, the crosses, the benches. It's a good system if you want to use lots of equipment. It keeps the session fluid and linear.

When I had my own dungeon I never used to clockwatch at all. I liked it so much it didn't bother me if we went over the agreed time. But now, because I rent a dungeon by the hour, I have to keep an eye on the clock. I hate it because I'd quite happily play for six hours if I could.

Each slave wants to go on a journey serving their mistress. Mouse's sessions won't contain any sexual involvement, but he has watched me actually having sex with a Body Slave so he has experienced the torment of that proximity without any touching. He likes to receive the marks of his mistress. It's like a trophy they can take home with them. Daphne's happy when his arse is still glowing weeks after I've caned him.

I'm confident in my own abilities, but the general rule is that most guys want to get an erection, want to come at the end of a session, or not be allowed to come by being brought to the edge on a number of occasions and *then* come right at the end, or be brought to the edge several times and then come when they go home to their wives.

Sometimes you get the guys who don't want that. They want you to torment them as much as possible but they're determined they're not going to get an erection. Although it's what they want, I feel that I've failed if I don't spoil it for them and give them a hard-on. I'm trying to get their senses going.

Sometimes they don't come back to me because I don't visually fit their bill. If you want a brunette, or a Chinese girl, or a redhead, I'm not going to work for you. They usually come to me if they like the way I dress or they've seen me on TV, or read good things about me, or seen one of my reports on the internet. If somebody wants a quirting they'll come to me because I'm the best there is with that particular whip. It doesn't disappoint me if I don't flick someone's switch. There's always the next guy. That's the nicest thing about it. Variety.

Some slaves want to test their own tolerance levels. If I get whipped I'll say don't stop till you cut me. And then when I'm cut I'll want more anyway. It's a delicious bright pain that's very compelling. Everybody tests everybody else, in all walks of life. I'm a bit of a cow because I like to test men in relationships too, push their limits, see if they'll crack. I know it's wrong, especially if they love me. It's stupid, because you can lose people that way, but it's in me. Do they love me or the persona? I always worry about that.

A lot of slaves like the verbal side of it, this art of being shitty to them. Rooster loves it, but he says I always take it too far.

From Slave Twin's journal:

Mistress writes:
You will be punished without a safe word.
400 x cane
2000 x quirt
cbt
Electrics
Slut training
Anal training
You will only drink water on one day to be chosen by me and your pain will be a rainbow. You will learn to obey me and you will suffer, Slave Twin.

Thursday
My nipples are almost healed. Still cut where Mistress's nails dug deep.

Friday
Danced, dressed and performed in pain. Tied and pegged balls and cock. Exquisite. High heels, straps and hanging chains. Mask. Earring. Ballet of torment. Imagined Princess my audience. Masturbated at end on knees, pulling leash to balls. Exhausted ...

Saturday
When we got home Mistress did not waste time in reducing me to subjugation and I was soon naked and, for various misdemeanours, she was going to cane me. She had me bent over and I wanted to receive my punishment with devotion, I was

growing to enjoy my punishment. What I like is how Mistress is always very strict about dishing it out and always gives me more. I received fifty and then another fifty for my recalcitrance. On top of that another twenty for moving. I took them all as I had to and when she had finished my bottom glowed with heat and I was in this amazing place where I felt so devoted and subservient to her and I wanted to fall on the floor, prostrate, and lick the soles of her shoes.

Sunday
I pegged my cock, balls and nipples as instructed and lay spread-eagled on the bed, the weight of the duvet pressing down on the pegs, twisting them. I wallowed in the slow prolonged pain thinking of my Mistress lying on the sofa, so far away from me as I suffered in silence, as my cock grew aroused so the pegs bit deeply. I wanted to endure it for Princess Spider and then she texted me and permitted me to come. Sticky and wet, I slept.

When a client comes to you for the first time, he must have belief in your skills, even without having previously sampled them. Remember, it is a big decision for a man to decide to take the step of visiting a dominatrix and proffering his naked flesh for punishment, to allow himself to be broken and turned into a submissive creature. So looks, and attitude, and ability are key. Trust is essential for any relationship to work, and it is no different once the clothes come off and the kowtow position is assumed. A potential slave wants to see his mistress in a pose of regal, even ethereal, majesty. He wants her to personify the things that in life he is in thrall to: power, beauty, danger, love. He wants someone to exude enough confidence for the both of them. I am certain I can provide the statuesque, almost physically overpowering, object of his need. A warrior, an Amazon. For a short time, I transcend what it means to be human. For an hour or so, I am his fantasy, his dream, his nightmare. I'm unattainable. An angel, a demon. I'll open the door and he will cower, no matter his size, his wealth, his social standing. He'll not be able to meet my eye. His voice will tremble. I will, in the moment of our meeting, utterly crush him so that he knows where he belongs in the pecking order – so very, very low – whenever he is in my presence. But he *wants* this. He wants to be able to give up the power and control that he enjoys or endures during his normal working day. I have to meet or even exceed his expectations. Within minutes of those first impressions, he will be kneeling in a dungeon, nervous, maybe even fearful. I need to have nailed his acceptance of his subjugation to me, but he needs to know that he'll see daylight again. It's a tasty, heady brew. You have to get the balance right. If he doesn't trust me, I probably won't see him again. So I mustn't break the golden rule and do anything psychologically or physically damaging to him, especially if he has expressly forbidden it in his list of dos and don'ts. His trust in me must be balanced by my responsibility to him. It is an essential synergy. We need each other in order to feel alive.

Session report by a debutant:

Eventually, after some time, the moment came and I answered the call. I was given directions to a location Mistress had specified and was required to call her on my arrival.

I think the moments just before meeting your mistress for the first time is an exciting part of the session, and an important one.

I arrived at the destination so I gave her a call. She wanted to know what I was wearing, so I assumed she was observing me from a nearby location. I described what I was wearing and I remember her saying 'Ah yes', as if she was accepting me into her world.

She then told me to turn around and walk back the way I had come. She gave a command to stop and turn 45 degrees to my right. I was then asked if I could see a spider, and there it was, the door knocker on the front door. She told me to make my way over to the house. I knocked nervously on the door and it opened. Princess Spider was standing there, dressed in PVC. She invited me inside. She looked better in real life than on her website, which is saying something.

I entered and we chatted about inconsequential things for a while. I was asked to make my way down the stairs into the dungeon where I paid my tribute to her. I was ordered to strip and kneel down. Mistress then slapped some cuffs onto my wrists and ankles. I made the mistake of turning around and showing my backside to my mistress. I was immediately corrected and told to rethink my position. I finally sat on the floor with my legs stretched out in front of me. Princess Spider then picked two objects off a shelf and asked me what they were. I said I didn't know. They turned out to be the rubber ferrules from the tips of walking sticks. These are squeezed onto nipples and give a good sensation when removed, sucking the nipple out to an extraordinary length.

I was then blindfolded, and told to make my way over to the table in the corner of the room. I did this very slowly, which turned out to be a mistake. I got a hard slap on my behind even before reaching the table. I was told to hurry up. I laid myself down on the table with my hands above my head.

The first item I found myself being introduced to was a cock ring, which was slid down my penis to the base. I also felt two rubber strings that were wrapped around my testicles and tightened. This was a really nice feeling and made me go semi-erect. After the cock ring had been fitted I felt a pinwheel being run up and down my testicles and cock, and then all over my body.

This was followed by hot wax being dripped over my flesh, and once again, my testicles and cock were most sensitive to this. My cock was twitching all the time this was being done.

While the wax was being applied Princess Spider fired questions at me: 'What is your favourite position?'; 'How did you come to like this fetish?'; 'What is your favourite colour?'; 'Have you ever served another mistress?' So many, so quickly I could hardly concentrate. I answered the best I could as my mind was on another planet. I felt I was already enjoying this session far too much. I could feel a rubber dildo being run over my own cock and testicles, and down towards my anus. She placed it to one side and said: 'This will end up in your mouth later.'

Princess Spider asked me if I had ever heard of her Inferno. I told her I hadn't, but that I would be interested to know more. Without a moment's hesitation I could feel a cool liquid being poured into my belly button, shortly after this I felt the small drips of wax being dropped onto my stomach, each drop moving nearer to my belly button. Just at the point of reaching my belly button, a river of wax was deposited on me. I could feel this river pour into my belly button and erupt. The heat was almost unbearable. The pain faded away quickly though and I found myself wanting more. Princess Spider slowly covered me in wax and after a short period I felt an ice-cold object following the same route. The combination of heat and cold being slid all around my body made me shiver with excitement. I was shivering so badly at one stage Mistress asked if I was all right. I replied that it was nervous excitement. This nervous excitement continued for at least half an hour. I eventually got my body under control.

I could hear her moving around beside me. She said, 'This is my dildo, do you think I cleaned it since the last time it was used?'

It was shoved under my nose. I replied, 'No.'

'That's right,' she said. The dildo was traced across my lips. I found this very arousing and decided I wanted more. I angled my head so that instead of the dildo slipping across my lips it went into my mouth. I started sucking it off like a good slut. I spent a great deal of time on this, removing any trace of Mistress's special deposits. I enjoyed this immensely. Princess Spider pulled it away from me.

'You're enjoying yourself too much,' she said.

I then admitted what I had always known. 'I'm a dirty slut,' I said.

'Yes, I can see that.'

She asked me a question which put the fear of life into me. 'I have another sub upstairs waiting, do you want him to come down and suck your cock?'

I immediately froze. I didn't know what to say and even if I did I could not speak, because I now had a gag in my mouth. So I shook my head. The mistress kept on probing, encouraging me to say yes, but I wasn't quite ready for this environment, I was only a mere novice after all.

During the session Mistress kept threatening to singe me and mark my body and also threatened to remove hair, but I had to refuse every time. There is always another day.

In the middle of the session Princess Spider started lightly striking me with a whip made of artificial grass. She used it on my cock, testicles and stomach. This was very enjoyable. I think I could have taken it a bit harder but I was afraid to ask for it. The gag was taken out of my mouth and I was allowed freedom for a short while.

Mistress asked me if I had tried needles before. I had not, but was willing to try. I heard her unwrapping the sleeve from one of them. I felt the icy swipe of a surgical cleanser on my testicles and then she moved them around slightly to find the right point of insertion. She quickly forced a needle into me. Immediately I felt an enjoyable hot/cold sensation around the area of the needle. I liked it and would definitely want to explore more in this way. The needle stayed in while we continued with our session.

I could now smell cigarette smoke, and although I am not a smoker this smelt very nice and I was quite happy to breathe it in. With the cock ring in place for sometime now, Mistress started to pull it upwards slightly. She also tugged my cock and testicles quite firmly, I don't know for what reason but I think I started to leak from my penis and this was like a red flag to a bull. The next thing I knew, wax was being dripped over the tip of my penis.

She said, 'This will block your hole.'

And with my penis now blocked with wax, it was time to gag my mouth once again.

'Hold on tight to these,' she said, while plugging my mouth with her panties.

This was great. I had a pair of Princess Spider's panties in my mouth, I felt quite dirty, but that's a good thing for me. These panties stayed in my mouth until the end of the session, so I was able to suck anything from them into my mouth.

She asked me another question: 'Do you know what this is?'

I could hear a tin being clicked open, then she started to rub something on the head of my cock. I replied, 'Tiger balm.'

'Yes, well done.'

I had got it right. My cock was already on fire before this was applied. It didn't make too much difference to the feeling, but it was still enjoyable all the same.

I was starting to wonder about how long the session was going to go on for. It seemed the mistress had done an amazing amount of things to me since the session had started, and I never knew what was going to come next. She was now asking me to lift my legs up. This was so that she could slip a skirt on me, and she pulled the skirt up to my waist. I felt a right horny lady, I imagined myself standing up, slightly bending over and lifting up the skirt over on one side so it showed my buttock and a glimpse of my arsehole, whilst making a small groaning noise, teasing anybody that might be watching me.

Princess Spider asked me to move off the table, which I did as quickly as I could. I was then commanded to walk to the middle of the room and bend down on my knees. I did this and Mistress slowly slipped the skirt up over my buttocks, in a similar fashion to what I had just imagined. I raised my buttocks in the air. I was hoping for anal penetration. Mistress started to insert a butt plug into me, but the plug she used was too big and caused a lot of pain. She tried a smaller one but still I had problems accepting this. Eventually I was able to receive an even smaller one. This was poked in and out of my arse, and although this was enjoyable, it was not what I had hoped for.

The phone rang. Mistress picked up the mobile and answered it; it was her next client. She told him he would have to wait as she was having fun, and I knew how she felt.

She continued pushing the butt plug in and out for a while, and during this time I announced to her that I liked to give rimming. She was interested in this, and asked whether I had been rimmed by my partner.

I said, 'No, I have been deprived of this act.'

Mistress then asked me if I wanted to release my load.

I replied, 'No.'

She got me to say, 'I'm a dirty slut who likes to withhold his come from his mistress.'

I said it once but Princess Spider shouted at me: 'Keep saying it! Again: I'm a dirty slut who likes to withhold his come from his mistress.'

So I repeated this over and over again. As I knelt there on the floor, bottom up in the air, once again I felt the trickle of hot wax being poured down the crack of my arse. It got nearer and nearer to my anus, until finally it hit the spot. My cheeks clenched as the wax rolled over the sensitive skin.

Princess Spider asked me if I would like the handcuffs taken off.

I said, 'No, I'm enjoying myself far too much.'

She laughed. She then asked me to rise, and with this started to take off the handcuffs and ankle cuffs. During this period of comedown we chatted about the session that had just occurred. I told Mistress that it had been a great session and I had really enjoyed it. I was pleasantly surprised to find Mistress remarking that it had been one of her best too.

We discussed each item that had been used and which one I had enjoyed the most. She showed me a few other items that had not been used that she seemed proud to show off. Princess Spider offered me a shower. I accepted this and I removed the skirt I was wearing and used the towel to cover me. I then followed Mistress up the stairs to the bathroom. She showed me some framed photographs. The pictures varied from mistresses, subs during sessions, and of Princess Spider. The picture of the lady sub being tied up securely with lots of rope took my fancy. I took the shower and made my way back down the stairs to the chamber where I met Princess Spider again. While I got dressed we talked some more, and finally I made my way upstairs to leave. I shook her hand and thanked her for a great time and wished her a good evening. To top things off, I checked my watch to find I had been in session for two hours. I was one happy bunny.

At first I worried a little bit about causing someone pain, or injury. Even knowing about safe words – that a slave could end their sessions by uttering it, that this was a convenient safety valve – didn't help much. It's a big step to thinking about it, to picking up a weapon and actually using it on a person. I could kill somebody with the quirt, believe me. But the fear didn't last long. There's no great difference between the pain you get when a tawse strikes your flesh and a punch you get while boxing, or a tackle during football. It's over almost as soon as it's begun. Sure you might have a bit of heat or an ache afterwards, but the initial shock, the worst and the best of it, is instantaneous. You have to realise that this is what they're paying for. That sting, that thrill. The danger and the body's self-protection in the face of it: the balm that comes as endorphins are released. They want it. They need it. And I need it too. Switching is important, I believe, if you want to become a great dominatrix. How can a mistress who has never taken the cane on her raw bottom know how heavy she can lay it on for somebody else? Pain is a great leveller. I've seen big army brutes unable to take six of the best and puny little men wearing mistresses out. I play hard because I love it but also because I need to know about limits and pain thresholds. It's as important to me as knowing what a person's favourite colour is, or what food he likes, or the music he listens to. Pain tells me a great deal about somebody.

I know pain so well I sometimes feel as though I invented it . . .

It's true to say that a lot of role-playing goes on in the dungeon. It's really just a beautifully designed theatre when you come to think of it, with the mistress and the slaves who use it playing out tragi-comic scenes. We're all frustrated actors and actresses. And we're good too. We all assume roles at home with our families, or at school or at work. We slip between personas with harlequin speed. We know our lines and never fluff them. We follow the cues like pros, and love our close-ups. I'm an auteur, really. I write the scripts, set the lighting, compose the shots, direct my cast. I see it all drenched in glorious Technicolor through my eager eyes. I call the shots. I make the cuts.

I've never worried too much about how I might react to a particular situation. I just let instinct take over. There's no point in worrying if you find yourself getting horny while you're whipping someone's arse, or dripping wax over a muscular back. It's natural. You can't control it. You might as well just enjoy the moment and let it feed your next move. This work is as much about animal impulse as ingenuity with whips and paddles. You can't just stop a session if you become randy. I'm human, I respond to various physical traits and occurrences. There's nothing like the feeling of power you get when you see a big cock thickening because of what you're doing to it. And of course that's going to get you going. The slave and the mistress feed each other and feed off each other. The only difference is that I'm in control and the slave is paying to give up his or her grasp of reality and destiny. I've never thought too much about what this means in terms of my own sexuality. Am I gay, straight or bi? Well yes and no to all of that. I'm neither homosexual nor heterosexual. I'm sexual. End of.

Introductory letter to Spider:

You asked me to give you a brief idea of my fantasy. I am very ticklish. I imagine being spread-eagled and have you use your fingernails on me. I would love to worship at your stockinged feet. I dream that the knickers you wear on the Wednesday before my visit are still being worn by you on Thursday (and maybe even overnight). Then when you tie me down you take them off and wrap them around my face, all the while tickling me. I am really looking forward to visiting you, and I am 100% sub and genuine. Yours humbly, Keith.

From Slave Daphne's diary:

Night of the Cane
Maybe this should be called *Night to Remember* instead ...

I had been looking forward to this ever since my Princess had told me that I would be going to it, but I am getting ahead of myself ... I'll begin with events earlier that afternoon.

I met my Princess in town as arranged. More to the point she met me as I was standing there with my thumb in my bum and my brain in neutral. My Princess was laughing, clearly enjoying the moment. We had a coffee and I was told to remove my clamps, which was a very painful operation. I displayed my nipples to my Princess for inspection. We did some shopping for short trousers (I thought it was only breath that came in short pants ...) and went back to the house where my Princess prepared a superb meal. When we had eaten it was time to get ready and on with the schoolboy outfit, except that mine came with a pair of hold-ups. I was so excited and truly hoped that I would be caned that night. Little did I know ...

We arrived at the venue and I waited at the bar while my Princess did her social rounds. Before I knew it, my Princess instructed me to get in the boxing ring. This was not for three rounds of boxing but to give my Princess room so that she could give me a caning.

Just before the caning began, my Princess told me she was going for 1000 strokes. I leaned against the ropes, presented my backside and the caning began. As the strokes landed and I counted them I quickly became aware that this would be no ordinary caning. Each stroke was far more severe than any given to me before by my Princess. Also the number of strokes given in rapid succession had grown from 10–12 to 20–25. I was aware of no one else in that room other than my Princess as she took me to new levels of severity and pain during the caning.

As the number of strokes increased my backside felt as though it was on fire. What I was experiencing was something so very beautiful and my longing was for my Princess to be getting immense pleasure from what she was doing. We had gone beyond the half way point and had reached 600 strokes when my Princess called a halt as I was starting to bleed. The disappointment that I felt was not for me but that it had cut short the pleasure of my Princess and I felt that it was my fault. One thing that I was not aware of at the time was that my backside had been photographed and key rings made. I quickly bought two.

However, there was nothing I could do about my backside other than to clean myself up and then return to the proceedings. Afterwards great interest was shown in my backside and it was inspected many times over so that people could see the results of the expert handiwork carried out by my Princess. I think my trousers went down and up more times than a yo-yo at the world championships.

Then came the caning competition. My Princess had been barred from taking part. It was easy to see why. The strokes that were being given would have barely counted as warm up had my Princess been delivering them. She would have won hands down.

After the competition my Princess was much sought after by people wanting their backsides caned by the number one mistress. So with their arses presented and cane flying my Princess brought smiles to their faces and their cheeks turned red. There was one thing that I did notice and that is every time my Princess starts to play a small crowd gathers to watch. This never happens when anybody else is playing. I never notice it when my Princess plays with me because when that happens I may as well be on a different planet with my Princess.

Then came a moment I hadn't been expecting at the start of the evening. That was when Rooster and I were ordered into the ring with my Princess as referee. It was hard work as we did our best to avoid punching each others' gloves with our chins. I felt knackered after each round and as a referee, my Princess was very strict. As soon as we went into a clinch in order to have a rest she soon broke it up. At one point Rooster went down and my Princess straddled him and started bouncing up and down. At the first opportunity I went down too because I certainly wanted some of that. To my great joy my Princess straddled me and did the same. For some reason I was adjudged to be the winner. Maybe that was because I was either sweating the most or it was OAP concession night.

As the evening drew on, we wandered into the area where the stage and items of furniture were and my Princess commanded me to get into the stocks. The elation that I felt was overwhelming, so down went the shorts and pants and into the stocks I went.

As I stood there waiting for my Princess I suddenly felt myself being caned and I immediately started counting. The strokes stopped at seven but by the time they had reached two it was clear that it was not my Princess doing it. They didn't have that perfect touch that my Princess has. I could not see who was delivering the caning but I had a strong feeling that whoever it was did not have permission from my Princess.

Then a new stroke landed, and this time I knew that it was my Princess. There was, however, a difference about this stroke. What I had been given earlier in the evening were the severest I had ever known in my life but what I was receiving now eclipsed even that. There was no let-up. If anything, the strokes became even harder as the caning went on.

The caning continued and as the cane landed again and again the pain surged through my body. I hoped that all were watching and taking note because they were witnessing a truly expert mistress of perfection cane her slave who so desperately wants to serve her totally and give her extreme pleasure.

The number of strokes increased and so did the severity of them and the pain I was feeling. I didn't want it to stop but it had to. Apparently the bleeding had become too great. My Princess had reached 280 strokes and every one was a wonder to behold. As I was released I put my hand to my behind and saw it was covered in blood yet I felt so proud of it. My Princess had taken me to beautiful places that I never thought existed. I was informed afterwards that the dungeon monitors had been about to call a halt to proceedings anyway, which was a pity because 120 more strokes would have meant my Princess reaching the magical 1000 for the evening.

By the time I had cleaned myself up it was time to go. At the beginning of the evening I had done as every slave would do which is hope for everything but expect nothing. What I had been given far exceeded all my hopes and wildest dreams. I had been given the severest caning of my life and I was proud of the marks I had been given.

As I write this my thoughts go to what awaits me in my punishment book. There are, at the moment, 1350 strokes of the cane due, not counting any additional ones that may be added due to further offences having been committed. As this is classified as true punishment and not just play I have an idea of what to expect as a result of this Night of the Cane.

A few weeks later ...

Thursday
I spent most of the day down by the river because when in the shade there it was about the coolest place to be. I had taken a book with me but it was difficult to concentrate on it as my mind kept coming back to the 800 strokes punishment I am going to be given in two weeks. I am looking forward to the time when I will be in the presence of my Mistress but those feelings are also filled with trepidation about the punishment to come.

Friday
The evening at the club brightened up when my Mistress arrived. I was so very happy to see her. As far as I was concerned, she out-shone everybody else there. During the course of the evening I was able to have a chat with my Mistress and she showed me her new cane. It didn't take much intelligence to realise that 800 strokes would be painful. I talked to her about this but as soon as I spoke I could see from the look on her face that I needn't say any more. My Mistress had already decided that once again she would be going for 1000 strokes. She told me that she wanted to do this and it is something I hoped for despite realising I would be taken to a level I didn't even know existed. Will my punishment be continuous or will I be given a break in the middle? Will the 200 extra all be with the quirt? Will my Mistress actually stop at 1000 or continue? I have never heard of anyone receiving 800 in one session, let alone 1000. So many questions that only my Mistress has the answers to as my

Mistress has the total right to do to me as she desires. As her slave I must willingly and gratefully accept all that she does. All I know is that it is going to be exceedingly painful.

Monday
I do not for one moment stop thinking of my Mistress. To say that she has total control over me is an understatement. She has complete control over my mind. She has me firmly in the palm of her hand. I received a text from my Mistress saying that she hoped I was thinking of her cane. I haven't stopped doing so since I first saw it last Friday night. I keep trying to visualise how strong the first stroke will be. The stroke that will set the pattern for the remaining 999 strokes of my punishment. My Mistress and I will soon be starting on a voyage of discovery. It is also a journey into the unknown as far as I am concerned. I was commanded to report in to my Mistress by phone. This will be done without fail as my one and only role in life is to totally serve and obey my Mistress. There is no other mistress who comes anywhere near my Mistress and I speak from over thirty years' experience, having met and 'played' with over sixty of them.

I love fucking at 4 or 5 a.m. when all is quiet and my Body Slave is sleeping. I listen to him breathing and he looks so at peace. I pull off the bed linen and slowly suck him to an erection. He stirs, I caress his balls and lick his shaft. I slip my nightie over my breasts so the cold breeze from the windows crawls over my skin; he loves my nipples to be erect. He is there to serve me, no matter what time it is, he must obey! When he has grown and his hard cock is in my hands I slide onto my Body Slave and slowly fuck him, sucking his nipples, spitting gently on him to wake him from his sleep then I return to his cock and taste him again, sucking and licking until I choose to mount him once more. I become more vigorous, sometimes slapping his face. I pound and scratch, I bite his nipples. I'm a scar in their minds and their flesh; I'm a wound they cannot heal.

CHAPTER THREE: SPIDER SKILLS

'The qualities I'm now using in business were in the background all along because of my Territorial Army training, and my father and grandfather being in the Army. I know about discipline. I had a fairly strict upbringing.'

Princess Spider

Dumpling's Homework: a fetish alphabet

A – Accept what your Mistress decides for you

B – Behave well at all times

C – Consider your Mistress with gratitude because she also knows that the letter C can mean cane or correction

D – Dungeon. This is Mistress's space and not your space. Mistress also knows D can mean desire for her

E – Expectation of your next meeting with Mistress

F – Forget your views. They do not matter. Mistress has removed them during the session and in her prior sessions

G – Genuine versus false. Mistress is the former

H – Honesty. Very important for Mistress in order for her to continue going forward with the necessary education. Very important for the subject because it took a lot to make the contact with Mistress in the first place

I – Intuition. Mistress's secret weapon. Very astute, very street cred, very tuned in and turned on to your needs. No underestimation of Mistress is allowed

J – Just desserts. Mistress will give you them
K – Kowtow
L – Look but do not touch unless allowed. Learn from your teaching
M – Mistress and nothing else
N – No. This is a word never to be used. You must always answer yes
O – Obey
P – Princess. The best. End of story
Q – Question your Mistress and her training methods? Never
R – Remember Mistress is always in control
S – Submission at all times when in session
T – Trust your Mistress
U – Understand Mistress is on your side but ahead of you in the game plan
V – Value her at all times
W – Whip and Wonderful Mistress
X – the love she gives you xxxx in correcting you
Y – Yes, the only acceptable response, Mistress
Z – Zeal with which you seek to improve

Outside of the military and the gangster underworld, I'm probably one of the most tooled up women you're ever likely to meet. I have items here that can cater for every kind of physical need. I have things in my possession that can reduce the strongest, most powerful men to blubbing wrecks.

I'm a traditionalist. I wear a lot of leather when I'm out. Everything matches: coats, boots, bag, caps sometimes. I have a different look. I don't suffer fools. People see me being really wicked, slicing slaves up. I can use those weapons so well. It's a phenomenal thing to watch, a dominatrix with complete mastery of her weapons, in full flow. And it's the paradox. The idea of the angel with blood on her hands.

There's quite a bit of snobbery in the mistress world. What annoys a lot of mistresses is that I'll walk into a room and the masters will come and talk to me. I have such respect for men. Not only because I can torment girls and make them scream their pants off and get them excited and aroused, but it's because I'm a female. If a man was pissed off and they dominated it would be in anger. The mistresses can't see why these masters are interested in me. Once I had nine guys talking to me all about Agincourt. Mistress Devastation asked me if I was going to be talking to the boys all night, clearly jealous of the attention. We moved on to Napoleon and we were there for two hours talking about history. It's not all about the hard end of a cane. It's about networking, forming relationships, leaving an imprint of yourself in someone's head so that when they need a special kind of attention, it's you who leaps to the front of their minds.

I have always had an appetite for kinky sex. Where does this come from? I remember talking to Twin about this and trying to work out why I do what I do, but I couldn't quite put my finger on it. I guess it must have come through exploring sex. There's something nice about tormenting someone and then giving them a reward. It's like as a kid you're being naughty and you get a bollocking but the next thing you know you're being given an ice cream. I explore more now that I'm with Twin because he's as fascinated as I am. It's nice that he desires me as much as he does. Others have said they did, but they were just once-a-day men. Twin will take any excuse to get into my knickers. It's nice that he wants me like that. I never get tired of him trying to chat me up. And I also like how we slip in and out of the game. A man might look at his girlfriend's bottom a hundred times in one day but if I catch Twin doing it I'll challenge him. 'Are you looking at my bottom?' And he'll say yes, and I'll reprimand him, or he'll say no and I'll still reprimand him. 'Why not?' I'll ask him. You just trip them up like that all the time. We might be out shopping and Twin will step in front of me to get to the till, say, and he'll look up sharply, understanding the mistake he's made, and hang his head as a gesture of respect and apology. It's great. It's like a secret thing between us when we're in public.

I have an inquisitive mind. I like to explore all aspects of life. I coax all my Body Slaves to 'rape' me. I love the idea of giving my sexual power to them, the weak ones, for a short time. They all need me. I love to be submissive during sex and yet I'm pulling all the sexual strings really. I love to entice them with sexual fantasies; I let them have affairs with me in their heads. They all want to be my perfect slave. But they all fail because I have very high standards.

I like to talk about sessions afterwards. I suppose it's my military background coming through! After our first formal session in the dungeon, I talked with Twin about how much I used the cane, or how little. Usually I'll cane him about 200–300 strokes. I have a different fast drumbeat style that is quite popular. Or we might talk about how his training with the quirt is coming along – he's still getting used to it, so we didn't use it because his back was marked from a previous session. We thought the time we spent together was too short. And it was funny to discover that we were both quite nervous. I don't know why because I've dominated in front of an audience, of two or two hundred people, and never felt any stage fright. The tension had been building up before the session and had carried through to the actual session. We just discuss the different nuances of a session and work out how it can be improved next time. We came to the conclusion that we both prefer to play at home. It's more relaxed and we can walk around naked or wearing ropes.

PERMISSION TO SPEAK: Slave Rooster

'The thing about all the slaves that we share is a devotion to her. Adoration is a word I would use. She has an extraordinary thing that hooks you. The fact that she's a dominatrix is appealing, but she has something in her personality that

seduces you. It's a really weird thing. I see myself as quite level-headed, resistant to influences, but it's difficult to describe it. It's in her eyes, in her voice ... it's a sort of vulnerability perhaps. When she likes to be dominated – which is something I couldn't do, wouldn't do – there's the contrast, power and vulnerability. It draws you to her.'

It's important to command a certain degree of respect and even fear among your clients. I've had slave boys run away from me in clubs. It's all about confidence, character, charisma. I ran my own school club St Thrashmore's where I was a prefect and I stood up for thirty minutes, busking it completely, and played with all the naughty boys and girls. People like my ability to cope with a situation. I was a house Domme at Club Wicked for a while but I'd get a lot of people coming up to me asking advice. I also worked with security and the owner, helping to project the right image for the club. It's about bottle. Getting out, doing medical play in the club, for example. Doing the stuff that turns heads, gets people off their backsides, talking, becoming interested in the fetish world.

The disciplines and scenarios that are played out against the dungeon background are infinite. The only limit is your imagination. Here are a few of my talents. If you find yourself growing curious about any of them, get in touch ... and form an orderly queue.

Mummification

This is like a form of bondage, but it's also a form of smothering. You basically wrap a slave in bandages Egyptian-style or you can even use cling film, which doesn't have the same kind of evocative impact, but it's very nice, and produces a different kind of feeling. Some slaves like to be totally restrained, rendered utterly helpless before their mistress. It is quite therapeutic. It's all about being concealed and not being able to move at all. I find this one of the easiest sessions to do because you shove them in a leather sack and tie them up with criss-cross lengths of rope and they'll either have a hood or a blindfold and the sleep sack will have a hood so they are completely enclosed. A zip allows you to torment the genitals. I have been inside one of these leather body bags and, believe me, it relieves stress. With the aid of incense and grass your mind can slip into another dimension. Some slaves just like to lie in their mummy state for the duration of a session. It's a bit like being put under hypnosis, a time when you can relax and empty your mind of all its tensions and traumas.

They're very comfortable. They can drift off and it's like being back in the womb, secure and comfortable and warm. I might play them some music or talk to them, or play a pre-recorded story with horny bits ... or they could go for a different kind of sensory experience via a piece of electronic equipment that plays different sounds and fires strange coloured patterns into your eyes. They go off into their own space for the entire session. I don't have to do anything physical beyond watching them and checking their pulse occasionally. It's extremely relaxing for them. They can just lie there, listening to themselves breathing, and watch this leather-clad mistress pottering about until the session is over. I usually chat to them if they want it, and take the opportunity to clean up the dungeon a little bit. Other than straightforward sensual play it's probably one of the most relaxing sessions you can do.

One guy, Henry, he's a corporate accountant, he likes me to be head to foot in leather, a hood as well, a cap on top of that. I'm totally anonymous. And he likes me to rub myself all over his naked body. I'm basically smothering him for the whole hour. His big fantasy is to be raped anally but when it actually comes down to it, he can never take it. One day he might be able to, but at the moment he just likes me in my commandant role. He's got a special liking for my Russian holster.

Others like to be smothered in different ways. 'Queening' is where you sit on somebody's face so they can't breathe. I don't know where the term comes from, but it's quite popular. As is placing their face between your breasts. There's a surprise. I can only guess that it comes from breast-feeding, or an aunt who cuddled them too much when they were young.

A lot of people like cling film because it warms you up. If you're cold and you play, your senses just go out of the window. You're constantly thinking about the temperature, and how chilly you feel. Also, if you're getting thwacked with something, it's a hell of a lot more painful. The cold changes the way you receive pain. It's better to be slightly warmer than colder in a dungeon. Spanking, whipping and wax play on cling film is an unusual sensation too. It kind of spreads out and retains the heat so you're not absorbing it in just one location.

Anal training

Fasting is very important. It can be pretty grim if your slaves fail to do this. Sometimes it can be disgusting. Essentially it's about training a man to take bigger and bigger dildos, right up to the monstrous beasts. Men expand more than women so they can take them better than we can. I start them off on a thin four-inch dildo, half an inch to one inch in diameter, so it's tapered at the point of entry. What I normally do is make them buy some muscle relaxant, and they're asked to take some before they come to see me. They're nervous and I'll make them strip. I'll give them a spanking, something to warm them up, and then I'll bend them over a table or a bench and try them with the baby one. I'll wipe them with Savlon or witch hazel first. It pisses me off if they haven't shaved themselves before coming to see me because it's cleaner and more hygienic if they do. I won't use my strap-on, I'll just put on some surgical gloves – I'm often dressed in my nurse's uniform for this, it all depends on them but they usually relate it to a medical process – I'll play some music, get them relaxed, lube the condom and roll it down over the dildo and insert it.

There's a knack to it. You want to find the G-spot, so it takes some rummaging around. If they're not too heavily built I can reach under them and press up to help stimulate it. Usually you know you're in the right place because they'll have an erection. It's not just about taking bigger dildos – there is pleasure involved as well of course. But the slave wants to take everything you can throw at him. They always aim to be the perfect slave but they never can be.

You show them the big one and say, 'One day you'll be taking this, slut.' And they look at you with terror in the eyes and you say, 'But today we'll start you on this one,' and show them something that is just a little smaller. I keep teasing them like this, playing on their fears. I'm giving them a real headfuck because they think I'm going to ram this monster up their arses. Sometimes I'll get the big one and put a condom on it and say, 'Right, here we go, you're having this brute today,' and go behind them and I'll have the little one hidden in my other hand. It's a great trick and it really gets to them. I might use a dildo that's like a vibrator and it's got the controls away from the actual business end so that's a bit weird for them when I'm on the other side of the room manipulating their sensations. Or I'll say, 'I'm going to use mine,' and that really freaks them out because they're going to get fucked by Mistress's dildo. Sometimes they get to worship Mr Pinky or Mr Blacky ... my own dildos. I'll get them to suck them, sometimes while they're being anally fucked. That's a good one. I've got a good sense of humour so I like to humiliate them by taking the piss out of them. A lot of them won't have done anything like this before. A lot of men have a powerful vision of a woman in leather trousers, thigh-high boots, a leather shirt, a cap, a belt and gloves and they want to get on their knees and suck my strap-on. I don't know where it comes from, but hey, if they want to kneel down and worship my rubber cock that's all right with me. They want to be as obedient as possible.

Some are bi-sexual. They'll come to me if they can't get a

boyfriend. It's no big problem. It gives them a kick. The erections some of them get when you put a dildo in are unreal.

There was a guy at Club Wicked who had seen me do a medical demonstration – I was piercing a slave's nipples with surgical needles – and he saw how careful I was. He bought these clear Perspex dildos from Holland, very attractive. He had a great outfit. I give him ten out of ten. He was wearing flesh-coloured tights on his top and bottom; he had them on his arms and legs and head and was totally in a body stocking. It would have cost him a fiver at most and he looked great. He was totally clean shaven and he said to me he didn't want an erection, he didn't want me to touch his penis, he just wanted anal play. I went up and up in size to the monster and it just went in without a grunt. He absolutely loved it. I had him on his back with his legs wide apart as if he was in the missionary position. I had him on his knees too. He took it all ways. It was a really great experience for both of us. It really inspired me. He was one of the best.

Some guys have failed though. There was a guy called Ryan who was pretty disappointed that he couldn't take it. There are some who ask for really flamboyant sessions. Daphne, who you've read about, is a prime example. He wanted hard play with the cane, he never wants a safe word, he wants nipple clamps with weights. I put these clamps on him – not the ones with rubber stoppers on them, these are savage things with jagged metal teeth – and he'd be on his knees and I'd be making him swing them, causing them to really bite into his flesh. The pain must have been excruciating. Then he wanted the cane. His first time with me. He must have seen some mistress who doled out six at a time. But I don't. My average is around 35 in one burst. So that was quite a shock for him. It blew him away and that was when he decided he wanted to serve me. There aren't that many mistresses who can get you to travel to that kind of rarefied point, but I play on the dark side. I can take you to the brink.

CBT

The simplest method of cock and ball torture is to tie it up with leather lacing. You can do it quite tightly and watch the cock turn from pink to carmine to a lovely deep purple. As long as it doesn't go black you don't have to worry. Orgasms while tied up can be extremely forceful. They move on to leather restraints that can have weights hung off them. They can't touch themselves in these objects. That's the whole point. There a leather sheath with little metal spikes inside. So if they get an erection they'll feel pain because the teeth dig into it. It's like a little Iron Maiden. After the fourth session they're asked to wear a cock strap and wear it all the time if they can. I like to personally choose them, once I've gauged their size! They're taught to think of me by wearing it. CBT can be anything from having the pinwheel run over it, to nails scratching, to waxing, needles, slapping. Anything goes when it comes to a cock and balls. Sandpaper, singeing, wooden spoons … anything. It's one of the most popular things. You can do it sensually with clothes brushes and feathers. Or you can use soft leather gloves which gives a different feel. Their partners probably don't wear gloves when they're making love, so to have a leather glove grab your cock or balls gives you a real buzz that you probably don't get elsewhere. You can feed thoughts into them. If they like CBT, the chances are they'll probably like nipple play. There's usually a link between the two. You can put clamps on their nipples and lay them on their back and then pull them up, you can see their nipples lifting away from their body – it must be agony – and then torment their balls at the same time. The erections they get are unbelievable. To warm them up beforehand I'll use an oil, a fragrant Tantric love oil called Nirvana, which you can get in the States, which I'll rub over them. That smell will alert them to the fact that CBT is about to start. It's like Pavlov's dogs. You'd be surprised how much people can take. I can lace up a bloke's gear, attach it to a pulley system, heave down on it and the whole of his sex organs will bulge and lift, dragging him off the floor. Release and pull, release and pull. They're completely at your mercy.

Some, like Twin, like it if you do it in reverse, so his cock and balls will be intricately tied up and I'll have a leash attached to it and I'll drag his tackle back between his legs and torment his cock and balls from behind. He says this makes him very submissive, because he can't move, he can't see what's going on. And he likes me to get my strappy red shoes with a Perspex heel and platform sole and include it with the lacing, so they're actually hanging off his cock while his balls and cock are being pulled backwards. It's a big thing for him. I did it in a sexy sensual way rather than in a dominating way. It completely blew his mind. But again, it's all down to your imagination. That's the only limit.

It's one of my favourite things, I think. But I couldn't do it. If anyone messed with me as roughly down there as I do with them I think I'd go up the wall. They must be really in control of their pain, or completely mad. But they feel safe and confident when I'm doing it, because naturally I'm not going to permanently damage the thing that gives Mistress pleasure ...

Trampling

Foot fetishists like anything to do with feet. Twin had me in pink mules at Kinkfest because he likes the way my feet look in them. They stick slightly to the shoe as you walk around and it's kind of a dainty clip-clop-clip-clop ... they make you walk in a certain way.

Whatever shoes you're wearing, trampling is what it says on the tin. You're trampling on the slave. It's a bit like ball-kicking. You walk all over them. I wouldn't walk on anybody's front while wearing sharp heels, maybe a low stiletto or a chunky heel. But I'll walk all over your back in high heels. Or you can do it bare-foot, or stockings or tights, for a more sensual experience. They like to see your painted toenails over your balls and cock or face or chest. I probably wouldn't do a full hour of trampling but I'd mix it up with related fetishes. Smothering, perhaps. They are always particular about the shoes they want you in. Mules or stilettos. And they'll specify Cuban stockings. They know in a very detailed way how they want you. It makes for a very interesting wardrobe, anyway.

PERMISSION TO SPEAK: Slave Twin

'I have a foot fetish. I'm an artist and I have drawn a lot, concentrating on feet, and there's a lot of my interest in feet echoed in the history of art. But it's also symbolic. It's the ultimate humbleness, to bow down, go to the place that is closest to the ground and kiss somebody's feet. There's a sensuality also, which is also in hands, but not as much because hands are easier to get to.

'I like shoes too, but shoes are there principally to bring out the beauty of the feet. Women's feet are a powerful focus for a lot of fetishists. It's pretty common. In China they did it for 2000 years. I had an Indian girlfriend who wouldn't let me touch her feet. It drove me crazy, but her reasoning was that to let me touch her feet was to somehow demean myself in her eyes, to put me below her. She touched my feet though!

'If a woman is dressed completely and the foot or the ankle is all you can see it's infinitely more erotic than if she's naked, I feel. You go to a beach and see women in bikinis and there's so many of them they don't stimulate you, but maybe there's a woman in a skirt and blouse wearing strappy sandals and there's more mystery and the chances are more men are looking at her than anyone else.'

Golden Showers

People want pee all over them for several reasons. Men like to watch because it's connected to the privacy of the female act. Men can do it in alleyways, up against trees, anywhere they like. The way a woman pees is a pretty secret thing. It's almost sacred. Men rarely ever see it, if at all. Seeing it is transgressive.

And lying beneath a woman and receiving it, is one of the ultimate forms of humiliation and degradation a male slave can experience. It's the idea that's so powerful. Some men really love it. Twin adores being servile and he loves my feet, so I combine the two to dominate him. I will hold myself open and put my foot on his face so that my 'champagne' dribbles down my leg and onto his face. It drives him nuts.

Capture

Essentially a kidnap scenario. The slave has a passion for being blindfolded and manacled. I'll put a bag over their heads and rough them up a bit, maybe before suspending them from shackles in the dungeon and leaving them to hang as if they're in a really rough prison cell. I might even interrogate them too. Mistress can then creep up and tickle them, or scratch them . . . anything to give them a bit of a jolt. Just touching them can provoke an extreme response, a scream or a plea to be freed. It's not so much a fear of being beaten as the mind seizing up, not knowing what will happen next. It's role play. I might wear my commandant's uniform for that. Different types of guys like it, quite a few with military backgrounds, which is strange when you think that they might once have been in a position where their jobs would put them at risk of that situation actually happening.

Dog training

The slaves have already got a dog collar, so they're in that realm of fantasy already. But some slaves are really into the idea of being this obedient lapdog and go so far as to try to replicate the look. There's a kind of leather hood that you can get that has dog's ears and a muzzle. Once they're wearing that they just basically do the kind of things that a normal domestic dog would: sit, roll over, beg. I'll give them treats if they're good, and chastise them if they're bad. They'll eat and drink from a dog bowl. And you play games with them too. I might put out four bowls in the dungeon containing dog biscuits, chocolate, cereal and dog food. Then I'll order them to sniff out one particular food and eat it. But they have to do it like a dog. They also have to learn to walk at your heel. I'll have them on a lead and make them walk very quickly like a poodle, in that kind of mincing way that poodles have. I did that at a party once. I had about eight 'dogs' marching around, making them pee by cocking their leg. And there's so many of them swarming around, some of them were almost up the backsides of the other dogs, so you have to give them a little smack and tell them that no, that other doggy isn't on heat, behave yourself. It's very funny. Some mistresses – I haven't tried this yet – have told me that they've taken their slave dogs outside into the woods. They really take it seriously.

Anonymous slave musings regarding 'Sub Space'

'My name is irrelevant. My only role in life is to serve. Being a slave to the first TV presenter who is truly a lifestyle mistress is a privilege. Mistress takes great pride in the quality and accuracy of her punishments. A natural sadist, she gets genuine sexual pleasure from inflicting pain. Her signature is well known in the BDSM club scene. She attracts hardened players who deem it a privilege to suffer a public quirting. My own experiences confirm her to be someone in control who knows exactly what is required to illicit sexual agony, a zone of pain, endorphin release, nice thoughts, orgasm, and perceptual change. Many call it Sub Space, a personal space no one can enter.

'It is a strange life. It is my life. Some may think me a pervert yet within the BDSM scene people are who they can't be anywhere else.'

Some slaves, after a session, will undergo intense emotional or physical experiences. A huge release of pent-up feelings. They might cry or break down. It can be overwhelming for them. Aftercare is really important in these situations.

The first time I saw Daphne in a club, this was before I'd even met him, before he was even Daphne, he was being dominated by a mistress who had a sparkler up his arse. Which then fell out onto his leg and he still carries that scar. And because he's a pain slut she left him but another mistress made the point that he couldn't be left like that and went to pick the sparkler up. She burnt her fingers. I remember thinking, this isn't very professional. I might use a sparkler up someone's bum but if it fell out I'd make sure I put something on it, pain slut or not. The place wasn't exactly clean; he could have been infected. That's the difference between me and someone who is downright vicious. Some guys like that, but if you put the tactile, sensuous stuff in there as well it makes it better for them. If you're punishing someone and then they get a tickle, it really messes with their head. Everyone's different, but I just like the idea of beating someone up and then giving them a cuddle. It might screw it up for them, but I've never had any complaints.

Daphne has often been quite emotional with me. He's used BDSM in the latter years to cope with his illness. Up until now it's worked – having never suffered with that I can't imagine what the pain must be like, but I've seen my aunt go through it and it's pretty horrific. Because he has to deal with chemotherapy it's changed the pigmentation of his skin. Part of what they put in that tastes of blackcurrant. When I was a kid I loved blackcurrant. I was a real Ribena kid. I've always drunk it. Funnily enough, me not knowing that he was on this therapy, I decided he would have to drink blackcurrant as a punishment – I often choose different types of drinks or foodstuffs for the slaves to consume; part of the punishment is them not knowing what it is – and naturally, this really freaked him out. He was begging me not to but I was insistent he drank it. He drank it for a while until he explained the reason for his not liking it. So I said, you can drink it occasionally, or if you've been especially naughty. It became a bit of a joke between us. But in one session we were playing a medical scene. He was blindfolded and I put the blackcurrant juice in a large syringe and put it in his mouth and shot it in and it really shocked him. After that I didn't do it again.

Aftercare is really there to hopefully negate any serious emotional breakdown – which is why it's so important for me to know beforehand about any medical problems they may have. For example, if a caning enthusiast comes to me I'll advise that they be wiped down first with surgical spirits or witch hazel – not in Twin's case because I'd want him to feel it – it helps to toughen the skin. Although I made a mistake once at a club and asked for some white spirit ... that would have been interesting – we could have had an arse burst into flames. Spectacular, but probably not a good idea.

Then after their caning I'll give them another wipe which helps to soothe them and aids healing, especially if they've been marked. Emotionally, they can be helped with a cuddle – it's an amazing salve.

From my own experiences of being dominated and experiencing the build-up of tickling, scratching, spanking, being forced to do things, expose myself, kneel in strange positions, the whole gamut of torment, I still get a frisson of panic, of fear. Even though you know this person well, you don't know if they're going to bring in someone from the next room to inspect your body, or touch you, or force a dick in your mouth. All or none of these things might happen when you feel so exposed or vulnerable. It's the anticipation, not the physical stuff, that can exhaust you and lead you to be emotionally weakened at the end. And it's worse if they know you. They're more brutal if they know you. They know how far you can go. And they know how to torment you mentally because you might have discussed your fears and frustrations with them in the past. It really gets you on edge.

And the pain, when your endorphins are released, can be unreal sometimes. I've had some pretty severe whippings from the quirt until I've cried. But after I've got that out of me I feel so relaxed. Recently I went to the opera, and the calmness I felt there was similar to that I feel when I've had an endorphin release from taking a whip.

If you lead a stressful life you need an escape sometimes. When I asked Twin to beat me the first time he was a bit reluctant, but I said 'You've got to do it. If you don't, I won't stay with you.' It's absolutely essential that I am with somebody who can dominate me. Once he did it, he was fine, but he had to get over who I was, what my reputation was as Princess Spider, in order to feel okay about it. He didn't like the idea of whacking a superior mistress when he is himself quite submissive. Once he saw how much I needed it and enjoyed it, he was all right. But he, as a submissive, can understand my need. He's in tune with it. He knows the pull it has on you, the way it can take you over.

Afterwards your release can manifest itself in different ways. You might feel relaxed, or energised, or horny, or tearful. It's like being in session and you might have the most gorgeous man in the world sitting naked in front of you but he might be extremely boring so you don't get turned on. But sometimes they might be someone you would never dream of sleeping with, going out with, someone as far away from your type as is humanly possible, and bang, something they say triggers your imagination and you feel aroused.

Twin has allowed me to permanently scar his back with my quirt. Many men can't play as hard as that, not because they can't physically do it – some can – but because they can't be marked because of girlfriends or wives.

I asked Twin what he would do about his scars if we ever split up and he said he'd probably get a tattoo. I told him it would have to be some pretty damned elaborate tattoo to hide those marks ...

I got him on the spine once with a ragged nail. He was winding me up and I did it in anger. I really sliced into him and it hurt him badly. He gave me a bollocking for it, but I told him to stop winding me up or I'd end up shooting him. He said he'd rather be shot in the balls than go through that again. So that's the only scar of his that I regret; other than that he really loves it. They're like trophies for him. But he's quite tough. I get him to lower his balls onto incense sticks. He does it gladly.

PERMISSION TO SPEAK: Slave Twin

'The sexual element of BDSM is, for me, not to do with pain, but more to do with power and control. The pain is an enhancement of that. You have to suffer for this pleasure of the sight, the smell, the things you can't actually touch or have. Corporal punishment has a limitation for me. It can't just be about that. It needs to have a more sensual side for me. It's about suffering for something that you love or are in awe of and think is really beautiful and special. And being prepared to sacrifice yourself and suffer for it.

'It's a visual thing too. Which is why I don't like blindfolds, even though they're obviously an intrinsic part of the BDSM world. Seeing inspires me if what I see excites me. I'm a visual creature anyway – I'm an artist – so I process a lot of information that way. I'll wear a blindfold sometimes because it's all part of the fun. I much prefer a verbal blindfold, you know: "Keep your eyes shut!" I like to give up control, but keep a little bit back. It's about my imagination, really. And it's the submissive, although they've given up the power, they're controlling things because they are the ones with the limits. The thing about Princess Spider is that she doesn't really pay much attention to what your limits are! Nobody's ever marked my back – and I've been doing this for nearly thirty years – except her.

'I'm not 100 per cent into being a 24/7 slave. The reality of life doesn't allow it. Some people want to be into that kind of thing. Some want to drift in and out of it. One of the fantasies I have is fucking somebody and not being allowed to come until they permit it. It helps stop me coming. I like the idea of great sexual experiences where you make out for hours, lots of *kissing, touching, but you don't actually climax, because an orgasm is the end of it. It's the getting there that's the fantastic thing. What I call "longing and lingering". When you have sex it's boom-boom-boom, over in seconds. If it's long and drawn out it becomes a control thing, it heightens the sexuality of it.*

'*I worry sometimes about how what I might ask for in session will reflect on me. I might ask for someone to beat me, or treat me rough, but that's not really how I am, it's just something I want in the context of an SM relationship. I could never treat a person in that way or be abused in that way myself. But within the parameters of play, it's entirely acceptable. It's a great feeling to go there and do what you want, what you need, and know you won't be judged, have people say, oh, that's what kind of person you are. Sometimes you do study yourself and think, "Is there a beast in me?" and there probably is in most people, but it's also important to be level-headed and to know that you are playing.*

'*I've never really felt self-conscious during a session. Not even the first time. There might have been a nervousness there. Do I really want to do this? Why am I here to get my ass kicked? Maybe I'm here because I just want to kiss her foot. You put yourself into it because you want to be there. And you've paid your money so you might as well get your money's worth.*

'*The variations of people's kinkiness is endless. What's normal for one person is strange for another. There are some fucking weirdos out there. But I can't really judge them because other people would say the same about me. The great thing about it is that there's no age limit. There are young and old people, different shapes, sizes and creeds. It's nice that it transcends all that.*

'*For me BDSM is a big part of my life, but it's not the whole of my life. It's an important facet of my life. I wouldn't live without it. I want to have "normal" sex as well as have extreme fetishistic sex. I know though that for some people it becomes the be-all and end-all. They can't get any sort of sexual release unless there's something kinky going on. It's a potentially obsessive subject. You're looking for the thing, like a red patent leather shoe, that will do it for you. It's like distilling experience down into one potent image. If it's black or yellow it just won't work for you. You end up blocking everything else out. It's important to keep a distance. To keep play in one place and reality in another. It means giving up a lot of things in your life and becoming very singular and anybody who does that is going to become boring. What makes people interesting, and what attracts me to Princess Spider, is that she has many other interests. There's a depth there and it has helped to make a strong connection.'*

It's quite exhausting, conducting a session. I've got to concentrate their minds, and mine, for an hour, maybe two. In the old days, when Dommeing was more popular, I would do session after session and might do as many as four in a row. You would physically drop and fall asleep after that. Now I do two hours and I feel the same. I often wonder how clients can go back to the office, if they've nipped out for a lunchtime session, and not fall asleep at their desks. The euphoria and fantasy must get them through it.

I'll get them to write about their session in their book on the way home, so that it's still fresh in their memory, and will remain fresh in their memory for as long as they have the book. I also instruct them to give me feedback on a session via an email, text or phone call a couple of days after they've seen me. It's all a way to keep them hanging on my web.

How many people are out there who tie themselves up, dominate themselves? I know Twin does it. He will text me to ask if he can put himself in rope. I couldn't physically play with Twin any more than I do already. Every time I see him, we play. And then I think, what does it mean that they're asking for it even though I'm not there? It makes me wonder, sometimes, if he can put this thing in the box and leave it there for a while, not keep wanting to play. I know why it is to some extent; he's never met anybody like me before who has opened so many doors for him, who shares his fascination and obsession. He's got his perfect Mistress. Is this whole Mistress thing going to destroy it? Maybe the obsession can be too great. Benson certainly let things go too far. Twin isn't overly obsessed, but with us the sexual side of things is so heightened, orgasm is so powerful, that I can understand why he craves it. He said to me, 'You're like a drug. I have to have you. Whatever little bit it is.' Sometimes he'll phone me at night so that he can hear me talk to him while he masturbates. I'll make him get my red shoes and get him to do it over them while I talk to him.

PERMISSION TO SPEAK: Slave Twin

'The Mistress is put on a pedestal. She doesn't piss, she doesn't shit, she doesn't fart, she doesn't eat, she has no problems, she's basically a Goddess: perfect.

'But an imperfect Goddess is preferable to a perfect Goddess as far as I'm concerned.'

CHAPTER FOUR: IF THE STRAP-ON FITS ...

'Most guys don't want you in your leather gear. It's amazing what they want you to wear. I have one client who likes me to wear white bloomers for him.'

Princess Spider

Uniforms and costumes ... there's no real significance involved in them, beyond providing a kinky thrill, a sensual jolt. It's usually what the slave boys request. When they get in touch I'll ask them what they're into, what they like. And they'll say leather, PVC, nurses, rubber ... whatever. The range of clothing is dizzying. Flick through a fetish catalogue and you'll be blitzed by jumpsuits and transformer dresses, mini-skirts and thongs, catsuits and empress dresses, starburst tops, spanking dresses, tit-flash bodies, mandarin dresses, Chinese hobble dresses ... I could go on and on. All of it in amazing materials that cling to the body like a second skin. I love leather, and I think I look at my best in it. But others will have a fondness for something else.

If it's really hot I won't wear rubber because it's just sweltering, and it can restrict your movement. It's nicer to be free. On very hot days I'm tempted not to dominate because once I didn't feel very well and this slave came in wanting this all-leather anal assault. I said, 'Look I might be a bit woozy, I had a fall earlier.' I'm always quite honest with them, and he said, 'Oh Mistress, go and take that leather off, get into something you feel more comfortable with.' And in the end we just sat in the dungeon and drank tea and chatted. He's a nice guy, works in the city, but can't get much free time. He got a leather-clad mistress to kidnap him on the back of a motorbike once! The fantasies you can get involved with are endless.

I've dominated in the nude, or in flowery dresses, nurse's outfit, riding outfit. I like wearing military uniforms best because I feel more powerful in them. There's something twisted about a dreadlocked soldier, because when I was in the TA I had short blonde hair. A lot of people like me in leather and there aren't many mistresses who wear much leather, mainly because it's so expensive. I get mine from Holland, where it's cheaper. Twin's different. He'll have me in anything from beads to pink knickers, a towel, my birthday suit . . .

It's well known that men are visual creatures. They get stimulated by what they see. So what you wear goes hand in hand with that. I always search for trigger words when I talk to people. I won't ask them directly about stuff but I'll just wait to see what kind of reaction I get to certain words and that will give me enough to go on, to surprise them with something connected to that later. During a conversation I might mention stockings and there'll be a twinkle in the eye and you can tell what disturbs them. Once you've got that hook you can throw it into the mix and really have them dangling.

When I'm out, they're all around me. One will get me a drink and one will rub my arm if I've got to play. I never have to light my own cigarettes. It's simple courtesy, and the slave idea comes from that, from treating women properly. Being a gentleman. It's quite an old-fashioned practice. If you went to see a mistress in the '50s you wouldn't see a dungeon as it is now. It could just be a sitting room. They might be in high heels, white blouse, split skirt with a hint of stocking. They were more like disciplinarians in those days. My dad was always respectful to his mum, and I was to my parents. And I try to teach my kids to behave the same way. They can be a bit lippy but they know when I mean business.

Stage shows are an important part of my popularity. They're enormous fun to do as well. But they take a hell of a lot of organising. To do this in front of 50–100 people takes some nerve. Some mistresses are quite lacking in confidence, believe it or not. They're not like actresses. They can do it in a one-to-one session, but nothing as big as a stage show; they bottle it. I've always enjoyed stage shows. I've done submissive demonstrations with Master Alex and once you've done that it's quite easy to switch to doing dominant because you've built up the confidence.

I brief everybody individually. I don't tell the whole team what's going to happen because that way I can use their mistakes to fuel the fire of the show. They need to make errors so I can do my job. That's what helps to retain the authenticity of a session.

Twin tries hard to be a good slave but he'll get here and I'll say, 'Where are my sweets?' and he'll have forgotten them. So I'll tell him to go out and get some for me. Of course, a part of it is that they misbehave on purpose, precisely because they *want* to get punished.

Kinkfest 2, London, July 2004

You step into the musty tunnels beneath London Bridge station, and you know you are in the right place. Petrol fumes and dust, the muffled roar of traffic and rolling stock. The great arch supporting the tracks and the trains swallows you towards an iron door on the right, where bouncers in black eye you casually. Inside you buy a ticket from the booth and move into Wonderland. The colours are black and purple, regal, mysterious. It's early, but already there are people swanning around in school uniforms, black leather, rubber and PVC, taking in the sights, sucking down as much visual candy as possible.

Through the hubbub and the smoke, a brilliantly lit stage plays host to Le Je Ra's *Re-animation*. A naked woman painted entirely in silver moves robotically, an android built for pleasure. She writhes and dances and, when introduced to a fellow droid, another alluring fembot, she is instantly attracted to her. Their creator is appalled, this is not what he had in mind. He wants them both to worship him. But together the robots overwhelm him and escape to an uncertain future together. The thrill of life comes from not knowing what will happen next. The slave world in microcosm.

The stalls are alive with curiosities and the curious. There are little displays and sideshows going on all the time. A scaffold is used to winch up tightly bound volunteers, their bodies awash with knots. You'd never believe rope could be so aesthetically pleasing. It twists and turns around buttocks and breasts, parting and exposing and lifting parts of the body like the very best supportive underwear. The girls turn on their fetters like gorgeous cuts in a butcher's shop. The flash of lightbulbs as photographs are taken. The hush of a crowd rapt with skilful rope magic.

You can buy clothes, ceremonial swords, kinky furniture, books. Anything goes. In dark corners, men are caressed, or spanked. Women are bent over tables to demonstrate floggers and whips. In a clearing, a man manipulates a giant bullwhip with the sensitivity of a lover, curling the vicious tip around bodies tense in anticipation of a violent blow that never arrives. A woman threads needles through the soft skin of topless models; purple silk wound around the steel to give the illusion of flesh as clothing. Electrical equipment surges and sizzles against naked bodies, evoking the black and white films of James Whale.

A corset is laced so tightly that it must seem the woman inside it will be cut in half. She glides elegantly away, her waist size perhaps as little as 12 inches. Stunning models stare down at you from fetish photography adorning the black walls. The roar of the air conditioning and the thrash and thump of music drowns out much of the conversation. It's a heady fascinating ride of the forbidden, the profane, the fantastic.

Back on stage Gwendoline Lamour performs a brazen burlesque – all tassels and teasing – giving way to the risqué songs of Rosie

Lugosi, PVC-clad vamp. And then the lights go down. You find yourself unable to breathe, as if every lung in the room has sucked all of the air up in one gasp. There is a surge as the audience move forward, as if as one. Cool blue light picks out a slave in kowtow position isolated at the centre of the stage. The skittering of music, like something spidery, flexes thinly from the speakers. Another light, a subdued alien green, tumbles upon another prone form. Out of the gloom a shape is coalescing, an ice-white mandala, enormous, pulling at the attention of the audience like something awful locked in race memory, something that demands focus and fear.

A giant spider's web.

More pale light. More slaves. All in poses of deep subjugation. You can almost see their heartbeats trembling under the naked skin. Slave Daphne, Slave Strangeways, Slave Vixen and Slave Nicky. Onto the stage comes Captain Clit, trainee of Princess Spider, the final player to make an entrance. The music changes and Spider glides across the stage to marshal Daphne and Strangeways into position. As she begins to warm them up with the cane, she orders Vixen and Nicky to remove their tops so that Captain Clit can commence nipple torture on them, trapped on the strands of the web like unfortunate flies.

Spider flits from her cringing male slaves to her writhing females with lithe athleticism before bowing to the public's hunger for her ability with the quirt, her weapon of choice. A jaw-dropping display ensues, Spider jinking this way and that, matching the rhythm of the music as its beat thuds and clatters around the auditorium. The quirt dances in her hand as if it is alive. The slaves jerk and arch as its fiery tongue darts against their flesh.

The lights dim and the darkness fills the creases of every mind. How long before they are able to think of anything but the spectacle they have just witnessed?

I actually dominate or discipline more women in club scenes or scenarios, but mostly in the school genre. On one occasion myself and the school matron went on a knickers inspection at a club. Most of the men and women present were willing to hand over their partners for a quick spanking and a tease ...

I have a female slave of the Web and she is very obedient and loves my torments. Female subs are usually more responsive to sensual play; their bodies are very intriguing to watch as they quiver under the tails of my prison cat. They especially enjoy candle and ice play; and I prefer their total submission. A female slave would serve me in more tactile, gentle circumstances. Having a women obey your every sexual fantasy is a truly elevating experience.

PERMISSION TO SPEAK: Slave Rooster

'It's interesting to watch her dominating another woman. It's much gentler, more erotic. But still powerful. She has the ability to get women eating out of the palm of her hand. The female slaves – and there aren't too many of them around – get huge pleasure from her.'

On the whole, though, although it seems otherwise, male slaves don't require sexual experience, they wish to serve Mistress totally, be it a maid service or total domination scene. The 'tied and teased' element is there, and most male slaves enjoy a varied scene or session on approval into my Web. They seem to appreciate the discipline factor of servitude and are more visually stimulated. They are very courteous and polite and respectful. I have met some deeply interesting characters. Men tend to enjoy the mind-power exchange that evolves in their sessions; they want to shed their work stresses and life problems, a kind of release from responsibilities for a short while.

Bisexual tendencies, in my case, help me to understand both sides of the lust coin. At the moment I have a heterosexual swing to my life; but of course there are times when a babe fires my Spider cylinders, whether it is a sub or dominant woman. I will always enjoy that side of my sexuality.

On the whole, though, my favourite experience is dominating a powerful man, and slowly bringing him under my control.

PERMISSION TO SPEAK: Slave Rooster

'A lot of powerful men – and I would consider myself to be a fairly powerful man within my field – like to be able to relinquish their power and be told to do things, rather than tell people what to do. It's quite a nice feeling.

'We were in Vegas, the two of us, on business. We'd done this whole day's shooting and we were both very tired. We were in a fantastic double room in the Flamingo Hotel, looking out over Caesar's Palace. We got back from dinner absolutely bushed. I was looking forward to a good night's sleep. One of the things I used to do for her was wash her knickers. We'd had a bath together and she threw her knickers at me and told me to wash them. All the time there are these little play comments, things like that. She went into the bathroom, I thought, ostensibly to brush her teeth, and I was lying down on the bed. Face down, drifting off. She came out of the bathroom and I had my eyes closed. She put a blindfold on me and tied me up and the next thing I know she's got her quirt out. One thing she does effectively is confuse you as to where she is in the room once you've had your sight taken out of the equation. Which then puts you in an anticipatory state. I'm not quite sure where she is and suddenly she'll touch you, or say something, and you think you know and suddenly she's somewhere else altogether. So you submit to the whole thing and decide to enjoy it, otherwise it would drive you insane. I heard the crack of her quirt and flinched because I know she can be very vicious with it – she never drinks when she's about to use the quirt because you've got to have a high level of accuracy – and she started lightly thwacking me across the arse and I was screaming a bit – they must have heard us next door, God knows what they must have been thinking – but it was *absolutely fantastic, just in that situation, those circumstances, in a hotel in one of the great cities of the world.*

'*It's what she says to you sometimes. You do end up submitting to her. It's inexorable, inevitable. She's got the ability to control you in those moments. You let her have you completely. She's quite crafty the way she uses her voice, its different cadences. It's very soothing but also questioning and wicked and teasing and savage. She'll play with you. It gets harder and harder. She's got tricks up her sleeve that can send a man off the Richter scale. She knows every game. And once you have experienced something like that, it's difficult to forget it. It's like being with a different person all the time. Every day there is a new challenge, a new face. It keeps you on your toes.*

'*Viva Arania! She is a remarkable Domme. I think it's because it's in her soul. She's a natural.*'

CHAPTER FIVE: CAUGHT ON THE WEB

'I've got a photograph of me as a little girl with angelic white curls. You wouldn't think this pretty little thing would turn into something that men have fantasies – or nightmares – about ...'

Princess Spider

It is the dead of night. I can't sleep. I need to unwind and there's only one place where I feel truly at home, where I can relax and find the peace I need. In the darkness I move through the house until I reach the simple wooden door. I unlatch it and sink into dreamland. I know where to put my feet instinctively. I know these smells, the ghosts of vanilla and jasmine incense. Of rubber and leather. Of blood and sweat. Fear.

Here is the glass cabinet with its cock rings and butt plugs and glass dildos, specula and electrical paraphernalia: the violet wands and TENS units.

All around are the soft gleams of padlocks, hooks, penis weights, the teeth of things used on nipples and genitals. Ropes hang around the room like guts strewn in an abattoir.

Here are the canes, paddles and rattans, lined up bolt upright like soldiers awaiting inspection. The thud of them against flesh. The intense heat. The skin can become raised with horizontals of pain. You can leave this place looking like a tiger.

Here are the equestrian whips, the crops, stingers and beloved quirts. They'll bruise and stripe your skin, cracking against it like distant gunfire, with tails that can cause cuts.

Here are the multi-tailed whips: the floggers and cats. Floggers can warm the skin, they can be quite sensual depending on the material used. They'll bring a red flush, as if your bottom were blushing at the attention it is receiving. Lines will come if the action heats up.

And the single-tailed whips: the Bullwhip. Stripes, welts. The daddy. Concentrated agony and an afterburn to last for days.

The walls seem to pulse with the memory of lashings and pleas for mercy.

The hoods and masks on their hangers stare blankly at the floor, even now, uninhabited, assuming postures of subjugation. The St Andrews cross waits patiently for another pair of arms to be splayed against it. It knows the tremble of bodies so intimately. The bondage throne. My place of rest. I sit there and take in the medical chair with its black sprawl of breathing equipment slumped in a gleaming cradle. Pulleys and beams. Leg spreader bars. Chains turn slowly as if moved by the ghosts of pain sluts visiting this place in their sleep. The metal trolley decked with sanitary wipes and boxes of needles, rubber gloves, swabs and a yellow sharps disposal box. Gels and lubricants and ointments. Syringes, mirrors, glittering anal probes. Cages. Candles. Cushions. Chairs and tables strategically carpentered to allow access to the most sensitive zones.

It's a Gothic laboratory out of Victor Frankenstein, it's the diametrical opposite of Sleeping Beauty's silk and satin boudoir, it's the ornate creaking door to a curious mind.

It is me, and I am it.

My heart beats as if, on the other side of that door, a slave were waiting patiently for me to permit admittance to his deepest nightmare, his most wondrous dream.

Preparing a dungeon before a session is a critical part of my job. On the day of a client's visit I'll get up and potter around in my nightie for a few hours. I'll have a long bath, with some nice oils poured in so that Mistress smells nice, and then a few hours before a session – it depends how many I've got booked, it could be as many as four or five, or it could be just the one – I'll make sure everything is hoovered and cleaned; I'll swab it all down with sterile wipes and then I'll switch on all the portcullis lights. I lay out dog collars, cuffs for both feet and hands, and a hood. I make sure all needles are stowed safely in a sharps box, and I'll select the essences I want to use – vanilla, jasmine and so on – depending on my mood and the particular flavour of the session coming up. I'm effectively turning this rented environment into my zone, my own personal sanctuary. I want that smell to help me find my own headspace. The music helps too. I'll light candles, and polish mirrors because the play of light in them can alter the mood spectacularly. Candles are also good because they exude atmosphere and I never know if I'm going to be waxing somebody.

I'll sit for a while in my dungeon, relaxing, thinking, meditating, taking in the ambience, finding some connection with that unique layout of furniture and equipment, and then very quickly I'll go and put my gear on. I always have a quiet time to get myself into that zone. It's almost like tunnel vision.

I ought to have a brief from them to read which they'll have sent to me previously: their dos and don'ts, allergies, bad experiences, previous mistresses. Sometimes I like to get on my knees and pray just before a session. I put me as Mum out of my head and think only as Princess Spider. I let her persona come shimmering through.

Friends will tell you that I can go up to the bathroom as one person, get my make-up and clothes on, and come down as someone completely different. I've changed, and not just in sartorial or cosmetic terms. If I go out I'll always put a pair of sunglasses on, even if it's night, because it's a part of my image to have this commandant or prison guard's look. It's important to have that private time before an event, because I can drift off somewhere else and find the calmness I need to operate.

Now I have to travel to work because I no longer have my own dungeon so I have to go by tube and walk. I'll have my spank belt in a handbag, and I'll leave an outfit in different dungeons, or I'll take something along with me that's much skimpier than usual because I've got to carry it. Dungeon equipment is always laid out. You walk into a fully kitted room. I'll be wearing my belt and they'll knock on the door and I'll be sitting on my throne when they enter. The throne is usually positioned so that it is facing the entrance. You want to be in their line of sight as soon as they enter. You want to be their immediate focus.

I'll ask them how their journey was and they'll give me their tribute. Then I'll make them strip. And then they must get on their hands and knees before me with their heads touching the floor. Without fail, every session starts like that.

They come into the room and the aroma hits them. It could be mainly incense, or leather – my old dungeon smelled very strongly of leather because I had so much of it – or an industrial smell. As soon as they get into that environment it's automatic that they get into their role. You can only tell when they're really relaxed when they've got their collars and cuffs on and they've given you their confession, or homework, and I'm reading it and commenting on it and picking at them. Maybe I'll put them over a stool with the threat of fifty strokes. And I'll know how cold a slave is because I'm looking for their reaction. I always say to them, put your head in the right place.

An example was a slave boy who came over for a two-hour session and just before he arrived he had a row with his wife – they were divorced, but they'd had an argument about children – and I said, 'You're not the same as usual tonight. What happened? Something happened. Do you need time to relax?'

He liked to drink in session and, although I don't approve of it, don't usually allow it, I know he can take it, so I got him a whisky. He had his girlfriend with him, she was waiting in another room, and she told me that he'd had this bad phone call five minutes before they arrived at the dungeon. I said, 'Don't worry – I can relax him. Give him time.' He was fine after that. He just needed a breather, and it was important of me to learn about this, otherwise I could have started punishing him while he was in this tender vulnerable state, and that could have been extremely damaging. You have to know your slaves, even the ones you've never met before. You have to have a little savvy where human nature is concerned. Being able to read people is a great skill in this business.

I give them a ten minute cooling-off period, maybe because the journey was hellish, or it's hot and sweaty. So I'm being a carer. You can tell how the session's going to shape up after ten minutes or so. It comes with experience. I can spot if they're going to be agitated.

Playing with Twin, more often at home than not, is different. We still use candles and essence, but it's something that can kick off at any moment. It's electric, unpredictable. We could be watching TV and I'll suddenly say to Twin, get on your knees and lick my feet. I have a habit of doing that. He's got to be ready at any time. He could be cooking in the kitchen and I'll grab him by the throat, push him up against the freezer and say: 'I want bottom worship,' or something like that. There's a list of things I'll suddenly demand and the best way of confusing a guy is to give him three or four things to do. Once they start cocking up you can feed off their mistakes.

Along these quiet back streets of Gravesend you walk. Behind the unassuming door in a row of terraced houses, you pass along a hallway decorated with mirrors and framed prints of beautiful women wrapped in leather and lace. You have ceased to be who you are from day to day as soon as your foot steps over the threshold. Your real name means nothing now. Now, you are Slave Rooster. And the clock is ticking. You know she is down there. You can hear trippy music beating through the floor. You can smell the incense. Your senses are on fire, straining for input. You can almost hear the sizzle of wax on the wick as it burns. You can hear her breath as she exhales smoke, the infinitesimal creak of wood as she re-crosses her legs on her bondage throne. You can feel the tension building in that crucible of torment, smell the rubber as it becomes beaded with moisture from the heat, hear the soft clink of chains turning in the air. You get changed into your leather briefs. You fasten the dog collar around your neck, with its identity disc pronouncing your slave name. It catches in the mirror and you are reminded who you are, what you are: *Property of Princess Spider*.

You descend.

She is seated, waiting for you. You dare not look her in the eye. But all the same her image burns through your retina like something branded there. At the bottom of the stairs you immediately sink to your knees and approach, head bowed. Your blindfold is neatly folded by her feet. You can hear her breathing. You can smell her perfume. She leans down low to you.

'Hello, Rooster,' she says.

'Hello, Mistress.'

'How are you today?'

'It's warm, Mistress. In the dungeon. It's a little warm today.'

She snarls: 'Do you think I care?' The voice suddenly teasing, honeyed. 'Do you have any confessions, Rooster?'

'Can I speak freely, Mistress?'

'Yes ... unless you bore me.'

'I masturbated once this week.'

She leaps on your words immediately. Nothing escapes her. 'What about the wank you had in my bed? That makes two. You will receive fifty for your fibbing.'

'I was excited in your bed,' you say. 'I couldn't help myself.'

'Did you wear my nightdress?' she asks.

'I wanted to, but I was afraid I would stretch it, or tear it.'

You gasp suddenly with pleasure and shock as she spits cold water over your back.

'Don't worry, Rooster,' she soothes. 'It's only rain. But not on your parade.'

'Thank you, Mistress.'

'Would you like some water?'

'I'm all right, Mistress, thank you.'

'What makes you think you're all right? You're in a dungeon with a vicious mistress. Do you feel safe?'

'Yes, Mistress.'

Laughter. She positions your blindfold and suddenly it's as if you're on your own. It's so still that it's as if she has vanished. You can't sense her presence anywhere, but you know she's there, watching you with that twinkle in her eye, that little smile curling her mouth. You are her experiment for the next hour or so. She likes to play.

And here she comes, playing now. You weren't expecting this: the smack of a wooden spatula on your backside. Cold wood, no give, the pain is excruciating. You begin to question yourself. You feel safe? Really? On it comes, the pain focused into that small space she's targeting with the spatula. Three, four, five times she hits you. The pain is everywhere and nowhere. Inside and out. You writhe and beg her to stop.

'No more, please. Please.'

She attaches a leash to your collar. 'Come on, puppy dog.'

Up onto a bench you go, face down, kneeling on padded rests, waiting for whatever she deems fit for you to undergo. The waiting is the worst thing. What will it be? The flogger? The pinwheel? The quirt?

The laval torrent of hot wax causes your back to arch involuntarily. You let out an animal groan.

'Do you know what your safe word is, slave?'

'Yes, Mistress.' But you don't use it. Not yet, despite the fierce heat of the wax. Because you embrace the pain. It's part of why you do it. You can take this. And you want more. The safe word can wait.

Now the pinwheel, providing a sweet stinging sharpness to offset the overwhelming sensations of the wax. Her strategies are almost as fascinating as the experiences themselves.

'Why are you being punished today, Rooster?'

Mind games too. Always the mind games. You have to be on top of it. You have to concentrate, otherwise she will have you so confused you'll be unable to talk.

'Because Mistress has had a hard week,' you say.

'Do you know your fetish alphabet, Rooster?'

'Yes,' you say, although you have never been taught it. It's another game. Another trap to fall into. Concentrate. 'A is for anal … B is for bottom … C is for cane … D is for dominatrix … E is for ecstasy … F is for …'

You should have seen this coming. Before you can say the word, you feel the bite of the flogger against your back. After a while, at the point where you are howling for mercy, she takes you down off the bench and orders you to lie on your back. She sits on your chest.

'I didn't tell you to stop,' she says. 'Carry on.'

'I is for invention … J is for jodhpurs … K is for kinky …'

Her fingernails score patterns across your skin. It's as if she has a map of your nerves; she knows where the zones exist that drive you wild.

'L is for love … M is for Mistress … N is for naughty … O is for …'

She moves, straddling your face now. She has removed her knickers.

'… oh my God.'

Later, she's using a feather on your buttocks. Things have calmed down. The brutality seems to be done with. She offers you gentle kisses. She breathes smoke into your face.

'Why don't you dance for me, Rooster? A sexy dance for your mistress.' You're happy to oblige. Now is a time for gentle play, for bringing you back to reality. Wrong.

She grabs you by the balls, twists you savagely, kicks you hard in the backside with a heavy leather boot. More with the pinwheel. More with the fingernails. Your nipples pinched, bitten. Endlessly innovative, the sensations coming so thick and fast you can't work out where you end and where she begins. And now the quirt. She twists it this way and that, moving it like a snake turning in the wind. Its bite is instantaneous, flying in from all angles. You drop to your knees, screaming out with the agony and the ecstasy of it all, groaning, squealing.

'What are you today, Rooster? A chicken? A pig? All these strange noises you're making. Carry on with your alphabet. I didn't tell you you could stop, did I?'

'No, Mistress.' Your brain fogging. Difficult to keep up, to know who you are, where you are, what is really happening to you. Concentrating on the alphabet brings you back to focus. 'P is for Princess . . . Q is for quirt . . . R is for roger . . .'

'Roger? Who's Roger?'

'Rogering, Mistress . . .'

That earns you a slap, but she's laughing too. She likes your humour, your playfulness. She forces you to lie down again. She listens to your heartbeat. You can hear a delicious unbuckling, the slow slide of leather as she eases off her boots. 'What am I doing now, Rooster?'

You hope she's putting on her shoes, the slinky ones with the enormous heel. Do you dare suggest this? What if she's standing over you, ready to mash one of those large leather boots into your face? You take the chance.

'That's right, Rooster,' she says. And you can breathe a little more easily. 'Now kiss my stocking tops. Kiss. Lick. Kiss. Lick. Come on, get that tongue working. Now the thighs. Now the shoes. Down to those pretty little red-painted toes. You may remove Mistress's shoes . . .'

And to the denouement . . .

She pulls your leather briefs down and swabs your balls with a sterile wipe. She swiftly pushes three needles through your scrotum. She twiddles their ends from time to time and you shift gently against the movement, enjoying the unusual sensations, the exhilarating sense of being invaded, of being impaled.

'Have you learned anything today, Rooster?'

'That it's not worth arguing with you, Mistress.'

'You may kiss my feet.'

'Thank you, Mistress.'

'Try to do better, next time.'

Body Slaves, rather than clients, tend to get addicted to me and my games. They get obsessed. They fall in love with me and then don't know how to handle life with me, they forget quickly that I am a woman, mother, carer, confidante. I'm a lifestyle mistress, and so I really like to play and torture my men; I like to take them to new areas of experience.

I suppose addictiveness in view of regular clients comes in the form of the endless phone calls from guys who just want to talk to me, but will in fact never come to see me, for financial reasons or family reasons. They crave to live out their fantasies but can't. I only take say five minutes of calls like this, then I will tell them to go away, nicely of course, or tell them to email me.

My ex-partner, Benson, was obsessive; he had craved, like Twin, to meet someone like me for about twenty years. They have similar traits. Benson would know that I had been in the dungeon on certain days of the week and he would return from work, bathe and then his ritual (they all have them, including me) was to lay out his fetish clothes for the night: a leather skirt, leather gloves, wrist cuffs, stockings, ankle cuffs, collar. After tea he would put them on and wander around all night in his new role as Slave Benson, the storyteller. He even worked from home sometimes in this outfit; I gave him the freedom to express himself.

I did not mind his obsession at first but as months turned to years, and we were not going out anywhere to straight functions, I started to dread him doing this, and would ask him to give it a rest. He did, but with a forced conviction. Sad, really, but I had to be cruel in a different way.

Some nights we would go to bed in our hoods and leather opera gloves and stroke each other or make love. This was nice and I enjoyed this experience with him. My hood is leather mesh like a fencing hood; soft and I can breathe well in it. I keep it at Twin's flat now. I have only worn it once with him.

Some men become obsessive by their jealousy. Body Slaves and partners they may be, but sometimes when all is over they linger on and won't let me go to live my life as I want to. I'm experiencing that now with Benson, he's hovering like a vulture, waiting for my Twin to slip up. But he won't and I love him for it.

I try to give all the client slaves specific days on which to email, phone or text me, 'reporting in' as I call it. This gives them the chance to give me feedback on sessions. Once a slave is named and is going to be a slave in training then they are committed to that regime. Their mind is not their own and they are to start at the beginning, a blank screen for me to scrawl all over.

Clients I don't like normally get me in my strict mistress mode. I will be very cruel and if they have bad body odour I will humiliate them severely. I'm quite happy to see clients that I don't gel with – it's nice to take your frustrations out on them – but if they are really obnoxious I won't see them again, or I'll really come down on them like a ton of bricks.

A slave I punished at Mistress Venus's place in Northampton was very disrespectful. I told him that if he did not show me due respect I would make him cry. I was told he hated singing, so I made him sing *All Things Bright and Beautiful* while he danced for myself and Master Ivan and Slavegirl C. He danced so pathetically that I took my quirt to him and gave him fifty. I knew he was testing me, he was trying to 'top from the bottom' (trying to be in control and direct things in the session). I stamp this behaviour out straight away. But still this slave did not call me Mistress when I asked him questions. I bent him over and gave him 300 with my cane and now he started to obey. There were now some welts on his bottom but at least his dancing had improved tenfold. He then admitted that he was aware of my superior teachings as a mistress but had not given him permission to speak. I decided I really had to teach him a lesson so I asked Master Ivan for his air gun and stood the slave up against a wall. I shot him twelve times in the balls. This helped subdue him but he was still being cheeky and lippy so I had to resort to the final punishment. I blindfolded

PRINCESS SPIDER: TRUE EXPERIENCES OF A DOMINATRIX

him, dragged him to his knees, parted his thighs and kicked him hard in the balls. I told him never to speak to me or any other mistress in that manner again. He cried and sobbed as I beat him to a pulp, dragged him over a bench and caned him again.

At the end of it all he grovelled over my boots and asked for forgiveness. Like a wild horse I had broken him, and Master Ivan was well impressed. The slave in question is now behaving well, being trained and lives with Master Ivan as a house slave.

I'm feeling ill, particularly rough, and it's late at night but I decide I need some fresh air. I ask Twin if he'll come out for a walk with me and so we set off, just a quick jaunt to the garage to get some cigarettes. While we are outside something happens. I know Twin and I know what turns him on, what kind of woman, what kind of shoes. And I know what I like in a woman too. And this shapely woman comes slinking across the garage forecourt in a Japanese dress and divine silver strappy shoes. *Clip, clop, clip, clop*, and Twin hasn't noticed her yet but I see his ears prick up at that unmistakeable sound. She's with her boyfriend, they've been out to pick up some pizzas, and they're strolling along the road ahead of us. Twin's very interested in her shoes, I know it, so I whisper to him, 'Imagine what those beautiful silver shoes could do to your cock. Come on.'

He said, 'What?'

I said, 'We're on a mission. We're going to follow them.'

All I've got on is my boots, my nightie, and his big coat over the top of me. No make-up. I feel and look pretty grim but this little escapade is helping to put a little life back into me. After a little while I decide I want a cigarette and ask Twin for a light. But he hasn't got one. He sees the little twinkle in my eye.

'Oh, no, Mistress ...'

'Oh yes. Go on. Don't you dare bottle it.' And I can see how he's watching this shape shimmer in the dark, how nice her arse is, and I know he fancies her. Hell, I fancy her too. 'Go on,' I say again. 'I want to see you suffer.'

I walk past the couple, who have stopped, and stand there leaning against the wall while Twin asks the woman for a light. I'm watching it all while she fumbles in her handbag. Watching his eyes, watching her eyes. And she focuses on Twin when she's giving him a light and I'm looking at her boyfriend and thinking, well, now she knows she's got a dish in front of her. Their eye contact is really good, and I'm enjoying it, I'm liking it. And he comes back to me and said, 'She's really nice.'

'I know, I can see,' I say. 'She likes you as well.'

We walk off in front of them and after a while we stop and have a smooch and they walk in front and they stop against this wall. I grab Twin by a fence and kiss him and I'm looking over and the guy is looking at me and I say to Twin, 'If I wasn't ill, I'd definitely invite those two back with us.' It was such a horny situation.

So on the way back I tell him, 'Tonight, when you fuck me, you're going to be fucking the lady with the silver shoes.'

'Okay.'

'But if you go sloping off to try to find her when I'm not around, you'll get at least fifty. Hard.'

Back at the house and I'm buzzing now. I've got the darkness in my veins. My blood is up and I want to be out there again with the moon and the stars and the wind. I want to be wild, not cooped up in this little flat. So I get dressed. Little short coat, leather trousers. Boots. And he's taking his clothes off.

'No,' I say, and there's something in my voice that makes him look at me. 'We're going out again. Put on your big coat. And bring the whip.'

We walk half a mile to the park. It's one o'clock in the morning. I get him up against the tree and I'm whipping him. Irregular strokes *thwit-thwit!* so that nobody *thwit!* can work out what the *thwit-thwit-thwit!* sound is. He's only wearing his trousers and shoes now. I'm scraping my nails down his back and I whip him again and he looks so great there against the tree, his broad back writhing and shiny, the muscles and tendons standing out like cords and he's really struggling because it's not my usual rhythm and he doesn't know when the next one will land. I kiss him on the back and he's hard and he wants me but I tell him we haven't finished yet.

'Put your top on, and your coat. And get your cock out. I want it to rub against the lining of your coat while we walk back.'

So he's walking back with this big solid cock rubbing against the silky folds of his coat's inner lining and he can barely stay on the footpath. Exquisite torture. I notice a clump of nettles on the side of the path and quickly grab a handful before he can see me. I pull back the flap of his coat and dink-dink-dink-dink-dink, I tap the head of his cock with these stingers. He's roaring. And his penis is throbbing and his eyes are watering and he's begging me to get rid of the sting so I tell him to wet his fingers and rub himself. But any moisture heightens the sting. I'm such a bitch. So now he's in real pain, the prickle of the sting and the luxurious rolling of the silk. He's still got quarter of a mile to walk.

Back at the flat he gets undressed and part of his cock has swollen to a ridiculous size. I take pity on him, command him to kneel and masturbate.

The secret is that it's not heavy pain. He can take much more, but what really reduces men to gibbering wrecks is the uncertainty. It was all gentle stuff – except for the nettles – and because I kept turning it and changing and teasing him, he was in pieces.

Every time I see Twin I want to punish him. It's a good foreplay to beat your man for six hours and then ravish him ... it works for me, anyway. He's always surprised. He'll say, 'My God, we've been playing for six hours.' And I'll say, 'Well, I haven't finished.'

He's never met anyone before like that. And I just keep getting more and more inventive. We just want to continue exploring. I think we're all like that, natural explorers. And with the BDSM crowd, you learn from each other. There might be a little trick you see that inspires or enthuses you and you're off on your own little tangent, pushing limits, trying out new things.

An early letter from Poppy:

I would like our first session to be a simple getting to know you as my new Nanny. Laying down the ground rules and you finding out about me: Poppy. I would rather be dominated by kindness than beaten black and blue as I am on my best behaviour when my Nanny is caring for me. But sometimes a smacked bottom is what I need, not all the time but just a way of keeping me in line if I'm very naughty. However, on occasion I do enjoy a little restraint, perhaps with shift reins, or being strapped to the bed so I can't fall out. I am aware of my own responsibility to look after Poppy in the sense of her being my inner child. At the moment a softly, softly approach would be appreciated.

Age play isn't a paedophilia thing, as some in the BDSM world would have it, it's about finding a safe place. If I want a safe place I'll go for a walk in the woods. For Poppy, it's getting into this role of being a baby, or a young child.

A typical session with Poppy would start with him arriving punctually. He's very good at that. His book is more about misbehaving or thinking naughty things on the bus while he was travelling to my place, so it's not sexual. Instead of kissing my hand or feet he will give me a cuddle. If I'm sitting on the chair he'll sit on the chair too or sit cross-legged on the floor. We'll have a chat about life in general, whether anything chaotic has happened in his life, is he okay, that sort of thing.

I would make him a drink instead of him making me a drink, which is what usually happens. Then I'll tell him to go to the bedroom and get changed. One particular time it took him an age to get changed and I was sitting there reading his book wondering where he was and he'd got into bed, when he should have returned to the living room. He'd climbed into bed. And you think, was he doing it on purpose, to be naughty, because of course that's what they do, so that they can be punished.

So he'll be in the bed and he'll have brought Whizzy, his teddy bear along with him – he usually brings teddies and toys – and I'll read him a story. Whizzy and the toys will all listen to the story too. He might have a dummy in his mouth, which is what he did when he first started seeing me, but he's 'grown out' of that now. He pretends he's three and a half so we can talk to each other. He's also in role as a girl during these sessions, so there are two things he's working on there. It's quite interesting that he chooses a girl's persona because it makes him feel safe. It's possibly because he perceives boys as being more aggressive.

He'll be under the covers and I'll make sure he's tucked in and that his toys and baby outfits are all tidy. I might bring my teddy Harry over and Harry can be quite naughty and try to get on top of Whizzy. Little disturbances with the toys goes on while I'm reading. It's fun. I'll interact with the toys sometimes, and they'll have a fight or something like that. It's not like some slaves who will purposefully disobey you so they can get punishment. It's more about me interacting with him. There's this maternal thing going on, even though he'll call me Nanny. We feed off each other. Stuff like Rupert Bear; I'll ad lib some of the stories and ask him questions about the pictures. I treat Poppy as I would any child of that age. It's quite nice because I always felt safe being Mum and having kids to depend on me and it's the same with the slaves and the age play boys. They all need me in a certain way. I respond naturally to that.

Then I'll put him down to sleep for a little while and we'll stroke each other as if I was his real mother. Occasionally he'll be naughty or cheeky and I'll lightly spank him, because he likes it. Or I'll ask him, 'Why are you wearing your shoes in bed?' It's a much more relaxing session than being in the dungeon. The dungeon has all those health and safety issues. You have to keep a check on heartbeats. But Poppy's in bed, completely safe, he's just got a handful of bears and there are no sharp objects to worry about. It's not sexual between me and Poppy. I don't get turned on, I just feel comfortable with him. Poppy sees me as someone who he can feel comfortable with. It's easy for me to switch between the roles of Nanny and Mistress.

On one occasion I had Poppy in bed and I was reading to him and downstairs I had two slaves beating the shit out of each other, taking my place for an hour while I read stories to Poppy. I had to slough off that Dominatrix skin, put a dress on and become Nanny. And then I'd tuck him in, say nighty-night to him, give him a little kiss, get back into the black leather, go downstairs and be very cruel. You have to have that ability to switch like that.

Poppy gets a sense of safety and security from a session. But sometimes he makes me very relaxed and he'll read to me. Sometimes he'll say he can't read a word and I'll help him. When he first came to see me he wore nappies, but it was just a comfort thing. He never messed them. Now he just wears frilly pants. Sometimes he'll wear a nappy in a club to puff out his knickers and emphasise his character. But age play boys come out of that zone pretty quickly, mainly because mistresses find it pretty offensive. Like anal play can be sensual and arousing, but disgusting if they haven't fasted beforehand.

I encourage Poppy to go to school events because there's lots of age play and transsexual elements going on there. It's good that he mixes. He hasn't come to a heavy session club yet but it will be good when he does – it's good because people sit and talk about why they're into things.

Being out there in the fetish scene as an age play boy takes some bottle. To walk into a room of a hundred and fifty people dressed as a baby when everybody else is dressed in leather, whips and chains. I think he gets strength, inspiration or courage from me. I encourage it because he's got to face up to it and do it if he wants to come out and be a part of the scene. We talk about it and what's coming up and I invite him to parties and clubs.

PERMISSION TO SPEAK: Poppy

'I started off as an adult baby when I was about 19. For a long time I kept it hidden. I landed up with severe depression – I'm still in therapy at the moment – but one of the first things my therapist got me to do was to accept this side of myself.

'My first entry into the fetish world was through seeing Mistress Fiona, who's retired now, and she really helped me out. Although I still have problems socially, I've opened up a lot. I think I probably am different from a lot of adult babies I've met online in that I'm not looking for a 24/7 relationship with somebody. But the thing I've learned from being in therapy is a lot of this adult baby stuff, dressing up and so on, is because I wasn't looking after myself in normal day-to-day life, so it's more a symbolic thing.

'My family background was fine. The only thing was that when I was very small we weren't that well off. Life was quite serious. So maybe I missed out on quite a few opportunities to just enjoy being a child. There was just too much focus on getting by, living day to day. It's not that I was abused or anything like that.

'The reasons why anybody gets involved in a fetish are complex. You can explore it, really get into the nitty-gritty of character and psychosis, or you can just say, I like to wear a nappy, or I like to be spanked. Just enjoying it. It's just an integral part of me.

'My interests have changed over the last few years from adult baby play to sissy cross-dressing play as well. Quite often people will come up to me and say, what do you like, what are you into? Having to put a label on yourself and say I'm a baby means I can fit in.

'The first knowledge I had about adult babies was in Forum magazine. It was that business of finding a couple of copies at the back of my parents' wardrobe, you know, and looking through the adverts about age play, there wasn't a part of me that said, this is wrong. It just flicked a switch for me.

'I didn't feel nervous at all, the first time I went to see Mistress Fiona. I had just been in therapy so I had had a chance to talk about it. I've been in long-term counselling discussing my development of relationships with people. I think that by building my strengths that way, adult baby play, as well as being fun, helped me develop as well. When I was 18 I was badly beaten up and my social life went to pot. At that time I was doing adult baby stuff at home. Going out and buying heaps of stuff, nappies, toys, plastic pants, and feeling very guilty about it. You go through this binge/purge cycle where you buy oodles of stuff, enjoy it, use it, feel guilty about it and throw it away. When my therapist suggested I explore this side of myself, I started building up a collection of clothes and toys slowly. It wasn't a case of getting everything at once and feeling bad about it. I've got maybe two boxes of stuff at home, but the thing is I might not get involved in something in public or private for months, and then I'll be really into it. I feel it's something I do, not something I am. I'm not saying that all people into this age play fetish are in therapy but in my case it really helped.

'It's something I use in tandem with therapy. It's not that every time I do it, it has therapeutic uses, but certainly there have been occasions when it's crossed over. One of the things I instinctively did as an adult baby was to buy myself toys and dolls and something my counsellor did with me – not knowing I had dolls – was to say, "This might sound a kinky idea but have you thought about getting yourself a doll to represent that inner child in you?" Which is what I'd done. When I'm relating to that doll as the child part of me, I'm very much the adult. It's given me a lot more control. I've met people who have been quite uncertain of who they are. It helps define me. It's important to explore these feelings.

'I met Princess Spider through Mistress Fiona. When she retired, it was quite a shock to the system for me, albeit a necessary one. It was upsetting. We were very good friends, but I asked her if she knew somebody she could pass me on to, would she do that? So she gave me Princess Spider's contact details. I was a little intimidated by Princess Spider because she has this reputation as a hard player, and she is quite a formidable physical presence, but there is a gentle side to her and I think there is a caring Mistress figure. Not what I'd defined Mistress Fiona, not the stereotypical nanny – although that's what I call them – they're not stereotypical dominatrices. I think it was a good step for me.

'If I'm going into character and acting as an 18-month-old girl and misbehave and get spanked that's not domination for me, it's punishment. It's a very definite division. I'm not into wearing a collar or serving a mistress – at the moment – but the relationship I had with Mistress Fiona is different to the one I have with Princess Spider. I think that a lot of the psychological care I had from Mistress Fiona I can now provide for myself. I don't just mean putting on a nappy and a frilly dress at home, I mean generally being better to myself than I was. I came from a background of self-harming. I think the fact that I've managed to explore these things has helped me.

'I can sometimes just watch a cartoon for ten minutes or suck a dummy for half an hour and that's all I need. Other times I get completely dressed up. But it's not to the extent where I was five years ago where I was constantly buying stuff from chemists and then throwing it away. It really takes over your life. There's an element of shame in it at times like that.

'There's nothing sexual in it for me. I can put on an adult-sized nappy and not get turned on at all. When I was a real baby, back in 1974, just before disposables were introduced to the market, I went from wearing terry cloth nappies and then switched over to disposables because they're cheaper. I think it's that feeling of being looked after, it's nice every so often to go back to it. It's good to call it age play rather than adult baby, because I'm not a typical adult baby. I'm not looking to be looked after 24 hours a day. Quite frankly it would bore me.

'I have brilliant fun with Princess Spider. We frequently end up in hysterics. One time she was reading a Rupert the Bear book to me and it didn't make any sense. We kept making silly comments about Rupert being on drugs. It doesn't need to be serious. It's a laugh.

'The thing that my therapist said to me – she works in a field of psychology called "transpersonal psychology" so it's very much dealing with spiritual experiences – was that everybody has a wounded inner child and yours just happens to be a little girl. I was actually terrified when I started talking about this that I might have a split personality. But it just means that I've noticed a part of my psyche and accepted it. That part of me was around when I was very small.

'The other side I've dealt with is that I was born in 1974 when corporal punishment was very much still a part of schools. I wasn't beaten a lot as a child – my parents never touched me – but I was smacked by a teacher. It was only once but it was very humiliating. I was about five and had a weak bladder. I put my hand up to go to the loo and thought she'd answered. Five minutes later I'm over her knee in front of the class being spanked. That really fucked my sexuality up for years. It's such a horrible form of abuse.

'I think I'll probably grow out of this phase, as if I'm reliving another childhood. There's this thing I do in therapy called two-chair work. I take my representation of Poppy as my doll and then swap places so Poppy becomes the parent and I become the child. After a while of wearing nappies it's boring. It's fun for a while, but you need something else to do.

'My role play age is about three or four, you can act up a lot more, have a conversation. But I'll probably move on. It's something I like to do. It's not just a crutch. I'll probably need to have the stuff around in some form, my box of toys and my frilly knickers, even if I don't actually use it. What I don't want to do is go back to that binge and purge state.

'The areas I'm interested in, TV and cross-dressing, aren't BDSM. It's not really my thing. I don't mind if Princess Spider *gives me a smack but if somebody else did it I'd probably turn around and thump them. There's a difference between spanking within the age play scene and people caning and whipping to get their endorphins flying, and that's great – but it's not my thing. I'm happy being me. I may not fit into any particular scene, but as long as people are happy and not hurting each other, that's all right with me.'*

I have a maternal side to me, a very strong maternal side, and sometimes, despite the whips and the gnashing of teeth and the angry bellowing, that will come through. If my slaves are close to me and I haven't seen them for a while, they'll thank me in the traditional way by kissing my boot and kissing my hand. Some of them will get a kiss and a cuddle. Daphne or Mouse or Freddy or Poppy will all get cuddles. There's a lot of tactile involvement, especially after I've whacked the hell out of them. I'll stroke the back of their head. A lot of mistresses don't do that. I'll always ask slaves, if they're wearing collars or cuffs, if they're comfortable. When they're in session and they're nervous, they perspire more. You've got to have water on hand for them to drink. The heat of the room can have an affect. They'll get a tender rub to reassure them. They're trusting me with their bodies. I like a laugh too. That can help to keep the atmosphere at the right level, or reduce the tension. I'll be caning someone, stop, and say: 'Does your mother know you're here?' You have to remember that if they're not happy, they won't come back.

I actually care about them. You often get a text asking if they can call you. Some of them want to unburden themselves of their troubles. You're a kind of therapy for them. I'm like an agony aunt. I like calls from the old boys who thank me for my time. Younger boys call and say, straight away, 'How much do you cost?'

And I'll reply, 'Do you mean my tribute?'

'Yes.'

'Yes what? Have you been trained by a mistress?'

'No.'

'No, *Mistress*.' And eventually, if they're interested, they'll start using the word 'mistress' and you know their head is in the right place. If they still talk to me as a normal person then they're not going to make an appointment and they're wasting my time.

I find European and American guys are usually more respectful. In my book I try to make them feel how gentlemen used to be. I get them to open doors for me, make cups of tea, light my cigarettes. I'm more traditional, despite the untraditional look. They have to kiss my boots or gloves, as tradition dictates.

The old fetish magazines prove that looks and clothes are really important. For some mistresses the penny hasn't dropped. They'll put a PVC dress on, buy a crop from a sex shop and hey presto, they're a mistress. But it's not going to be within them, running through their blood. Anyone can hit a person with a cane, but the subtleties that make that all-important difference just aren't going to be there.

No-shows and time-wasters are a real bane to the modern-day Domme. Have a look through the letters page of any BDSM magazine and you'll find mistresses belly-aching about these lowlifes. They ring your phone and the display reads *ID withheld*. That's how you identify, pretty conclusively, whether they are time-wasters. I've got this reputation now and they just want to ring me up and talk to me. Sometimes they'll call and they're not respectful, they don't call you Mistress, and you know they're just messing about. Or I'll give them my PO Box number and they'll say 'Yes, Mistress', and I'll ask them to repeat it and they can't, and I just put the phone down. I haven't got the time to entertain these jokers.

That said, I do have time for phone slaves, the genuine ones. I get them to send me money and then they can call me and I will speak to them for twenty minutes. Maybe I'll sit in the dungeon where there are rattles and shakes that they can hear and enjoy, and I'll recall a session I had with one of my slaves and talk them through it. It will be interactive, so I'll be speaking to them as if they were really there in the dungeon experiencing it. I'll get them down on their knees, order them to put on a blindfold and close their eyes. It's a poor substitute for the real thing, of course, but it's not bad as an alternative. A lot of men can't come to sessions for whatever reason – they're too scared, they're married, they're too far away, they can't afford it – so this is one way they can at least get a flavour of what goes on.

I had an Indian doctor in Scotland who used to phone me up from his GP surgery in between patients. And there he'd be on his knees, serving me down the blower while he had a waiting room full of sprains and headaches ...

I also get people who call me up who I've never met, never spoken to before, and they aren't exactly time-wasters, they just want a chat. I had a horny Frenchman call me and he was on the phone for half an hour, having a wank while he was telling me about how he was a naturist in London wanting to see me. He had such a horny voice that I thought, what the hell.

Basically, though, to show they're genuine, they need to send a deposit and a letter of introduction. If they don't do that, then I pay them short shrift.

I'm quite approachable. Some mistresses will look down on you in clubs. When I realised I was making headway in getting people to understand what it is we do, I was at Club Wicked's birthday party, and I was gaining a little bit of media attention and an older mistress came over to me and said she thought that what I was doing was great, it was giving the scene a boost and showing that we weren't all these seedy spank and wank types. There have been lots of little boosts like that over the years. If I want to commit myself to a project, I don't usually have trouble finding people to help me. They all want to be a part of the Spider's Web.

CHAPTER SIX: FANTASTIC VOYAGE

'I believe that I've lived before. I have a vision of myself as a medieval person punishing somebody. I know they must have tried to hang me because I have an affinity for breath play. And I've always had a stiff neck. That belief feeds what I do now.'

Princess Spider

Clients and erections. They go together like love and marriage, or a horse and carriage. It becomes very hard for them ... They want to stroke themselves. They look at me with lingering lustful eyes and the potency of my perfumed body aroma sends them crazy. They sometimes beg for permission to touch themselves and I might allow this, but at a price. Perhaps fifty with my cane or quirt or a nice leather paddle!

Many men have erectile dysfunction and they ask me for advice so they might solve their marital problems. Sometimes I can help. I plant a seed of lust, perhaps by getting a slave girl to lick their balls while I cane them. You'd be surprised by what can work. Mistress teases them and orders them to get big so she may enjoy looking at their cocks.

On their next visit they report improvement in their lovemaking with their partners, and Mistress's therapy has worked again ...

Many slaves ask for relief during or towards the end of a

session. This occurs by attaching a lead to their collar and then to a plastic dog bowl with a dog clip. They are then ordered to milk themselves into the dog bowl. 'Milking' is the correct term for sperm release in session.

A Body Slave would be milked by Mistress 'force fucking' them, perhaps while they are tied and lying down on the dungeon floor. I would climb on top of them and tease them into a frenzy, rising slowly from their manhood and pausing at the edge of their climax. Great for me, frustrating for them.

An old boy called Master Eugene, in his 80s, saw me playing at The Gate; he saw me caning a cock. Later I was talking to him, spiritually getting into the right place, and he said, 'Princess Spider, you really know how to play on the dark side.'

The dark side is not when you take pain levels beyond anything else, it's a place in the mind. It's about putting people in a special place. You have to think of nice things to cope with the pain. If you imagine yourself naked on a sunny beach, the heat infusing your skin, maybe you can hear the shush of waves breaking on the sand, then you won't feel the sting as much when the cane or the whip bites. As soon as you think oh shit, here it comes, you'll feel the pain. You have to play around with the mind and the fantasies. There aren't many mistresses that will do that.

I used to go to church every week when I lived in the Midlands. But when I got here I couldn't find an Anglican church. So I usually go to the Catholic service at Westminster Cathedral. It's quite ritualistic and the whole experience chimes with my own sessions which are quite ritualistic too. The candles, the music, the different light tones, that kind of thing.

My old dungeon had lots of different lights in it so I used to change the mood by flicking different switches, dimming or brightening the space, changing music, lighting essence burners. In this way the slaves would learn how the session was moving into better or worse territory, for them, maybe about to become more severe or sensual. I've always been like that and attending church has helped me to understand how mood can affect an environment and a person.

It started when my cat Sammy died when I was a child. I was gutted – and I've always had cats since then. One night I woke up and Sammy was sitting on the bed. I must have been about twelve years old. I could see him, as clear as day. I didn't bother moving in case he went away, I was just so happy he was there.

One night shortly after my dad died I got up to go to the loo and my dad was in the hallway. I said, 'All right, Dad?' and went back to bed. I see things. Sometimes I see the future.

Not many people know this but if I'm going to do what I consider to be a severe session I have to go to church. I always do that. It puts my conscience in order. Some of the things I have to do to men are quite severe so there's a nice sweet side to me to counterbalance all of this vicious stuff. I'm not saying I'm not happy with what I'm doing, because I am, but Twin says it's because I'm a typical Catholic. You do something naughty and you go to confess. If I don't go to church first I probably wouldn't do what I do.

If I've got a show or a heavy session organised I'll go to the church to get some energy. One time I was so tired I could hardly see. I went to church and prayed for about twenty minutes. As I was walking back through the church towards the doors, my eyesight began to get clearer, suddenly I was refreshed and I was ready to go. When I sit in church my entire body goes hot, which is also what happens when I heal people.

I believe in reincarnation. I was around in medieval times. I must have been to be such a wicked bitch! They tried to hang me, which explains my love of knotted ropes and mock strangulation. There's something in it. I'm convinced. It helps me with the character I promote. You can see the mystery in my look. There's a sense of a back story. A past. I draw power from it, and by God, don't my slaves know it . . .

Slave homework:

Out of the corner of my eye I watched Mistress come to stand beside me. Her tool was ready and big to punish me as only a strap-on can. She lifted and jiggled my clips and began to pull on my nipples. My body yearned for complete domination. I could not stop myself sighing with pleasure whilst wriggling my arse to draw attention to my hungry hole.

She responded by giving my arse a firm slap on its already red criss-cross patterns. The burning feeling spread through my bum and on to engulf my belly. Oh yes, I wanted to be an obedient slave to my Mistress in every frustrating desire. Again she slapped her hand down to engulf my smooth buttock in flashing pain, and then, oh so gently stroked my other cheek. Laughing, she told me how she would hate to see that cheek neglected and she followed up the gentle stroking with another hard resounding slap. The more I was slapped, the hotter my bum became and the more I had to wiggle my hips. My arse felt as if it were bouncing with pleasure and pain. My penis felt full and yearned attention from this dominant woman. I could feel the glans was wet with pre-come.

Moving to kneel behind me she slid her gloved leather hand up my inner thigh and groin to hold my balls in her hand. I was twitching in anticipation to receive her. The last of my inhibitions were forgotten when I felt, at last, the big full head of her strap-on rest against my flesh. Thrusting back I tried my best to engulf her but instead received a slap that made me squeal with frustration. Before I could recover I felt her magnificent length come gliding in. All it took was one thrust to fill me completely. She rested herself deep inside me and I could feel the head sending waves of pleasure through my bum and penis and belly. She began to saw in and out of me, building up speed, gaining in intensity. The pounding increased in pace and vigour and my rump was again given a good spanking.

This was beyond my dreams. I could feel myself rushing towards an orgasm. Her hands brushed my tender nipples as she continued to impale her devoted slave. Down my belly to my penis the black leather glove travelled. Her grip felt divine as she coaxed my penis and fucked my bum in such a teasing rhythm. I began to chant that my bum belonged to my Mistress. I love this woman.

Suddenly my penis jerked and my arse tightened its grip. I clamped down tight and held her inside as I came.

Thank you, Mistress.

I'm a Pisces, so fantasy and dreaming are part of my normal life. I think I'm something of a frustrated actress. There's a lot of fantasy and role-play in what I do. I frequently help slaves play out different scenarios with props and, occasionally, lines that have to be learned. In session, sometimes, it feels as though you are acting out a scene from a film or a play. It's pretty much the entire nature of BDSM. But it's second nature to me. I never feel self-conscious. I seek to explore as much as possible within my different careers: being a Domme, acting and writing. Sessions are real time, not fantasy, for me. It only becomes a fantasy when I mentally tease my slaves with visions, such as suggesting that they are being caned by a slave girl while they fuck me. That usually pops their corks!

I don't agree with that argument that fantasies die once they've been acted out. I don't consider it dangerous to pursue a fantasy until it's been experienced. Every experience gets better; I have just as much sex and love-making as I did when I was eighteen, probably more.

The other night we were all here, me, Twin, my two boys, and the boys decided to go down to the pub to watch the football and they were gone all of two minutes when Twin decided to drag me off to the bedroom and start playing. He was taking my clothes off and the next thing I know he's got the dressing gown belt around my wrists, a blindfold on and he's munching me, teasing, tickling and tormenting me and I'm thinking, 'Jeez, five minutes ago I was watching TV with my sons and now this is going on.' People wouldn't believe it. It's incredible sex, he's dipping himself into me and pulling out and teasing ... and I'm completely gone, at his mercy, and he's feeling around for my G-spot with his hand and he finds it and I bolt back, crack my head on the headboard and all the chains and whips hanging on the headboard come crashing down and I'm getting more and more entangled in equipment as he massages me and I'm exploding and I don't know where I am or who I'm with or what's happening any more. Totally amazing. Then we have a bath and nip down to the pub to have a drink. It's a different life and it can take me, this delicious madness, at any time.

My sex drive has never diminished. But my men are getting older and they can't keep up with my appetite. I have a strong right hand though, and often spend late nights alone wanking about fantasies of group sex. A fantasy always stays a fantasy in my mind, even if relived again and again. Excitement for me is the power of finding new secrets and turning them into recipes of lust, which I enjoy. I love to twist my words around their minds to give them visual stimulation as well as the mental aspects of their fantasy.

Twin, for example, has evolved his fantasies, so they still retain a flavour of what originally aroused him, but they have adapted to take in new scenarios, twists, adventures. His current appetite is serving as a Body Slave while being caned by a slave girl who holds a leather leash which is securely tied to his balls. He is being restrained, pulled away from between my spread legs, where his straining cock is millimetres away from my hot and ready pussy. It blows his mind!

Clients might sometimes feel ashamed of fantasies they have, or childhood experiences that have pushed them in sexual directions they might never otherwise have taken.

They all confide in me, sometimes when they cannot confide to people who are closer to them personally. There's one guy who I call my panty slave. He used to play with his sister's knickers when he was a child. I found that a bit weird at first. He used to rummage in the linen basket to get these used pants out. He was putting them on and sniffing them. This moved on to his girlfriends' knickers, which is, I suppose, more understandable. I get guys begging me for mine, so now I sell pairs through my website. It seems like a popular thing. He sent me all these pictures of panties and so, because he was a postal slave, I created a document all about knickers and what he should do – there was a picture of these frilly panties and a girl wearing seam stockings, and I instructed him in this document to kiss the picture, sniff the panties, and encourage his panty worshipping fetish. He bought a pair of mine for about £50 which he has to sniff every day and write about. He mainly keeps in touch by email.

Some of them are quite naughty. There was one guy, Philip, who comes to see me once a month – he hasn't been for a couple of months, I think he's been away – but he also sees this Thai masseuse and lady of the night. He tells me all about her because he has quite a high sex drive and he likes to experiment. His girlfriend or wife is quite straight in her sexual appetites, whereas he likes anal sex. So this masseuse will explore that side of things with him. He doesn't classify this as an affair, more as a release, but I suppose I would do the same thing, go to see a Domme or a masseuse if I craved certain things, and funnily enough in session with me, he never wants to get an erection, or to come or anything. I think he thinks it would be more unfaithful with me rather than the girl he has sex with. I don't know why, that's just his own twist on it. But I've had him close and after sessions he's told me it's been hard not to be hard.

This guy phones me up and leaves a message with his phone number. I notice it's an Orpington number. He says his name is Norman Ward. So I get around to calling him back and a woman answers.

I say, 'Is Norman Ward there?'

And she says, 'Yes, this is the Norman Ward. Who would you like to speak to?'

And I realise. And I think, should I put the phone down now or check it out? But I'm curious so I say that someone phoned me but I didn't quite catch his name. She says it might be someone called Leonard. So I ask to speak to him. He gets on the phone: 'Hello, Mistress.' Sounding a bit nervous and edgy.

'Where, exactly, are you, Leonard?'

'I'm in Green Park home in Orpington. I want to serve you and lick boots.' His voice is very shaky. He wants me to go there, but I say no, I want him to come to the dungeon at Camden. And I get Twin to drive me and hang around, just in case. He was a bit nervous about it in case Leonard turned out to be a psychopath and try to harm me. So I agreed that he could sit in the next room but with the door open because Leonard is probably in a place where the doors aren't shut or secured and I'll know by his reaction to the open doors how things will be.

I get there early to do the prep and I'm walking along the street and I see this short gentleman in baggy Bermuda shorts and a Walkman, gently rocking as he stands there on the pavement. And I'm thinking 'Is he rocking because he's looking forward to be beaten, or is he rocking to his music, or is he rocking because he's a psycho?'

'Hello,' I say. 'Are you Leonard?'

Big smile. 'Yes, Mistress.'

So I get Twin to go downstairs and put any sharp weapons away while I make Leonard a cup of coffee. I'm sitting on a chair talking to him and he's looking for his tribute and there's only twenty pounds in his wallet and he says that he's forgotten to go to the bank so he doesn't have his full tribute. He's getting a bit tearful but I get Twin to go to the bank with him. I felt he was no danger at all. He was more like a big child. So he collects the money and we go down to the dungeon to finish off our drinks. I'm dressed in very conservative clothing because I didn't want to appear too threatening to him the first time I saw him. I'm basically talking to him like a care worker. I didn't really want to punish him because I couldn't gauge his reaction to it. So I thought I'd just do an assessment. I started writing down what he liked: foot worship, licking boots, PVC, how he found out about me (in a magazine), why did he want to see me.

I asked him if he'd like to kiss my boot and he was happy kissing it for a while. And then we were talking and he said to me, 'Do you know, Mistress ... some people think I'm the son of Satan.'

I said, 'Do they really, Leonard? Who would say such a thing? You don't believe in Satan, do you?'

'I don't know, Mistress,'

'What do you think this is?' And I showed him a cross.

'It's a crucifix,' he said.

'Do you believe in God?'

'Yes, Mistress.'

'Well then, you have nothing to worry about. God is far more powerful.'

And he seemed to forget it then and went on about PVC dresses, which made me think that he had said it just to get a reaction, to try to freak me out. Being a naughty boy.

He might have been in his mid-thirties so I treated him like an 18-year-old who had been naughty but needed some guidance.

I said, 'Do you like it here?'

I wasn't sitting on the punishment throne any more. I wanted him in a position where he could see the door. We talked about football, all kinds of things. He told me he was in a home because of stress and that his family couldn't cope with him. He said, 'I'm glad to be here with you all day, Mistress.'

I told him he wasn't there all day because he'd paid for an hour and a half and had messed about so much walking to the bank and waiting there for service that we only had fifteen minutes left. He started crying so I told him he could go somewhere else before he went back to the psychiatric unit. I sent him off to Soho for a couple of hours of fun to have a look at things he wouldn't normally see. He didn't want to go back but I told him he had to and to call me when he got there. We said goodbye and I gave him a cuddle. It was a strange session, quite tense, and I felt I had to be firm with him when he mentioned Satan, but I never felt in danger. The owners of the dungeon were a bit uneasy about him being there but I said I didn't care what was wrong with him, he deserved a chance to experience something different, if that was what he wanted. I didn't even touch him. I gave him a hug, that was all. I made him feel that I was a sister to him. I reassured him. I haven't heard from him since. In one way I was frightened, but I wasn't. I was too worried about his own wellbeing to be really frightened. I hope he had a good time.

They're all conquests in a way, all good experiences. There might be some who have this strong desire to see a mistress and they'll ring me up frequently in order to talk to me but they won't make that final step and come and see me. They just want to talk about their fantasies. I don't know why they're scared to live them out, because I live mine out and they just get better, they evolve. It seems like a step too far for some, perhaps because they're scared or embarrassed. The ones that do bite the bullet and strip before me, they visibly shake, they're so nervous.

Sometimes it's difficult because a new client will turn up, such as Slave Alice, and they'll be in a bad state, really in a panic about the session. It's hard work to get them to relax to a point where they can enjoy the session.

Alice was telling me how he had never seen a mistress before. He couldn't explain what it was he wanted to explore, just that when he saw my picture he experienced this spiritual connection. I said it was strange he should say that from just one picture because I get that response from a lot of people who've been to see me a few times, but not really from a new slave. I suppose it was my eyes that did it for him, because the picture he saw wasn't a particularly intense dominating scene. He now has that picture in his punishment book. He's got this ornate mirror, over a hundred years old, with pictures of me around it and that's his altar of respect.

I will attempt to accommodate disabled clients whenever I can. I know a lot of mistresses will draw the line here, but physical needs are physical needs. The need itself is not disabled, so why be prejudiced? There's a guy called Allan, from Belfast, who saw the TV show and he's still saving to come and see me. He wants to have a session with me and a slave girl. He's got multiple sclerosis. He'd need to be carried down the stairs to the dungeon. He wants to be physically enclosed, covered up, so that his body was hidden. Which makes me think he's got some kind of physical deformity. I come from a caring background and know a little bit about deformities. I wouldn't say I've seen every kind of disability but I've seen a lot. It never shocks me. I often wonder how they cope. But I'm happy to see them. He wants a four-hour session – about £600 for me and a slave girl – and that's with a discount. I'll be happy to do this for him. It makes him happy and it could even help him with his disability. Everyone needs an outlet for their desires.

So they'll talk about things. They talk about family problems, or if they're gay they'll talk about how their relationships are or aren't working out, whether they've been bullied, how women didn't work out for them, how they're coping. I'm like a confidante. I've even listened to the infamous Dave Courtney's problems.

Dave's an animal. I got invited to a party one time and there was some filming going on. I was wearing a black PVC top and skirt and a pair of high heels. I had my first whip with me, right at the start when I was going clubbing. Dave walked in and I was sitting with my friend Gary. He was quite taken aback. Gary knew Dave was into fetish but he didn't know he'd be there. The party was great and I was sitting there with Baby Freddy and Dave said to him, 'You're in my seat.' Freddy didn't stand up at first so Dave opened his coat and there was this big silver gun, which caught my attention because I love guns and knives. Freddy moved then.

Dave started talking to me and he asked me if I wanted a drink. I said there wasn't much I liked at the bar but I was drinking brandy and Lucozade. He wanted to know what it was like so he bought me another one and he tried it and in the end there were two or three other hard nuts drinking brandy and Lucozade, which was quite funny.

We did some filming together. We were playing in the dungeon and Master Alex decided to dominate me. He got me over this chair with a Browning gun and it had a long-extension silencer, and he was actually fucking me with this silencer. He couldn't find my G-spot so I had to fake it, but I was faking it so good that Dave said, 'Wow, you're fantastic, you're like a really natural porn star.'

I said, 'Well, I'm not a porn star, I'm a Dominatrix.'

We were all playing around, swapping with each other. Master Alex was demonstrating with the bullwhip, getting it to curl around my body. I was down to my underwear by now. I was wearing a lacy neck scarf around my waist, which really accentuated my figure. I was slimmer then as well so I looked quite good. My hands were up in my hair and this whip was caressing my body. All the footage was going to go in Dave's film that he was making at the time, *Hell to Pay*.

Dave decided he wanted to stand me on a sofa in front of a great big mirror and put a truncheon up me from behind. That was quite exciting. I was screaming a bit and he decided he wanted to fuck me, so he did that from behind and it was great, my first fuck caught on camera. It was very erotic with the dim lighting and the mirror. It just seemed like me and him, even though the room was full of people. There was a good connection there.

After that Dave told me I deserved some fun, and he wanted a pussy worship scene in his film, so I'm lying there with my legs wide open, and I'm so thirsty I get a guy to toddle off and bring me a beer, and this slave with a bald head starts munching on me and half way through I just tip this lager all over his bald head and it splashes everywhere and it was really erotic. I didn't even consider where this film might end up. I was just enjoying the moment and getting on with it.

I found out recently from one of my phone slaves that the footage has actually been on the Bravo TV channel two or three times ... He rang me up and said 'Oh, Mistress, I've just seen you on TV and you looked divine, and it was very impressive what you were doing with that truncheon. Lovely to see you in your submissive role.'

What had happened was that it had been deemed too raunchy for Dave's film when he tried to get it released, so it had to be cut. Dave sold the footage to Bravo. Naughty boy.

A few months later, when *Hell to Pay* had been edited, we all went out to Cannes where it was shown, about sixty of us. I didn't want for money, there were loads of bodyguards, we went out to all these lovely places. He's got a fantastic sense of humour, Dave, despite his reputation as a hard man. He's quite vulnerable too, in many ways. I remember we were at this party, and he was sitting outside, and he was a bit depressed about something. I came out in my fetish gear and he said, 'Wow, you've made my night, you look amazing.' And he just wanted a cuddle. I found it bizarre. This great big tough man with all his tough entourage standing around him, and I just sat in his lap and he gave me a cuddle.

Before we went out we sat on the seafront and he was telling me how things were, what was pissing him off, what was happening in his life, and he said there was this one guy in his group who had been winding him up. He asked me if I'd come on to him and offer him a free session as a way for Dave to get his revenge. So I found out who the guy was and it turned out he was the owner of a club in London. I'd heard that he liked a bit of coke so I thought I could use that weakness on him in session.

We went to the club dancing all night, where I worked my magic on him, flirting, teasing, giving him some delicious verbal, came back and I went to his room. He liked nipple torture, apparently, but I hadn't brought any gear with me. Back then I was very worried about having to explain a bag full of dangerous goodies to customs. So I looked around and found some bulldog clips and some candles. I got him on his knees and started slapping him around the face. He was quite a tough guy too, so it was quite a kick for me to be beating him up. He said he wanted to give me pussy worship and I said, 'Oh yes, that's what they all say. But you have to earn it.'

I got him over the bed and was smacking his arse red raw. I didn't realise how thin the walls of the hotel were. All the boys who were there on bodyguard duty were in the rooms either side of us being very quiet, listening to this almighty commotion as I beat the crap out of this guy and, at his request, gave him a load of verbal humiliation. I was feeding him coke and champagne. It was totally debauched. I sat on his face and I was slapping his balls and I noticed he had quite a nice big cock so I thought, right I'll have some of that, and I put a condom on him and rode him like a horse. I had a towel around his neck and I was gripping on to it for dear life, and it was so vigorous that the legs of the bed came off, the bed crashed to the floor, the split bed mattresses slid apart and we sank in between them. We were there for three or four hours. He was totally blitzed by my appetite.

I had a shower, ordered him to clean the place up and got dressed in this lovely golden-brown evening dress. I prowled out into the hallway and heard this slow light handclapping behind me. I turned around and they were all there, watching as I made my grand exit. I said, 'Hello, boys, I'm ready to go out.'

Dave said: 'That was fucking fantastic.'

Dave's had a lot of girlfriends in his life and I knew I was one of many, but the difference with me was that I think he could genuinely talk to me. We'll be friends till the day one of us pegs it.

Some of the slaves that come to see me enjoy the complete withdrawal of any responsibility. The session and what it does for them is completely about them. They don't feel any pressure to satisfy a partner, or worry about their technique or performance. It's a complete ego massage. The consequences of that can be quite potent. One time a slave came to see me who was wearing a red PVC dress. I put him in a medical chair and blindfolded him. I usually make my slaves masturbate into strange receptacles. What happened to this slave this particular day, Slave Mouse, was that he'd been having a taste sensation session. So I'd been giving him little bits of chocolate, Bovril, bananas, baby food, maybe even pee, things like that to keep him on his toes. It's quite interesting to see their faces when they've been eating sweet things and you give them a dollop of Bovril. I gave him this thorough thrashing up against the cage, whipping him, caning him. I gave him a glass to wank into and he has a fairly big willy so it was quite a task for him. He was masturbating and I was tormenting him, twisting his nipples, spanking him, tickling him, talking seductively to him, scratching him, putting visions in his mind, as much pervy stuff as I could think of – which is a lot – and I could see him tensing up and getting faster and he gave this cry and started coming. He totally missed the glass and shot up the dungeon wall. In this particular dungeon the walls are lined with velvet . . . so it wasn't particularly clever. But I got him to clean it up. He was officially my Wallpaper Man after that.

Slave Alice has got this thing about pants – it's always pants or thighs or stocking tops – and he was wanking into this dog bowl that's attached by a chain to his collar. I was sitting on the cushions in this dungeon in Camden, relaxing, smoking, and I was getting him to recite the words 'I am a worthless slave' while he's pulling himself off.

I said, 'You're not looking at my panties, are you, slave?' He likes to be humiliated when he's coming so I was really abusing him. Sometimes when it's a nice bloke I find it hard to say disgusting things about them.

There are other guys that come to session and they don't want me to speak to them hardly at all. They just want to be punished. I sometimes think that when they don't want me to speak, they just want a whack, an orgasm, and then go. If there's no interaction it means they don't get to know me. They don't come back very often. Maybe once every six months, or else they're mistress collectors who like to build up a mental library of experiences with different women to refer to when they masturbate.

Wanking in session is quite common. Most mistresses allow it. Some will say they themselves don't have orgasms in session but I know that some of them do. It's a grey area, because I always maintain that pussy worship among Body Slaves in training is not sex, even though it obviously is, because it's within the context of a session and it is training a slave to be more obedient. It's difficult for a partner to accept that I have Body Slaves.

Sessions can bring the most powerful climaxes out of you. Some slaves don't want to come in session, they want to wait until they get home. Or they might make love to their partner while they think about what has happened at the session. It's funny but none of them think of it as betraying their wives, because, I suppose, there's no real sexual contact involved. Unless I say so …

CHAPTER SEVEN: PASSING ON THE FLAME

'Guys I dated nearly ten years ago keep in touch ... I must have something that touches their soul – I'm quite a spiritual person and they can't quite let go.'

Princess Spider

I'm still wondering whether my decision to pass on my knowledge to budding young mistresses is a wise move ... but if you've been to as many clubs as I have around Europe and in London, you'll have seen a lot of amateurish ladies. My decision to do this is triggered by the wish to see more safety within the BDSM scene. I once saw Mistress Fifi at Club Wicked whip Captain Zip with the straight end rather than the business end of a riding crop. That's plain dangerous; I found that quite disturbing. When I was the House Domme at the club I saw a lot of lifestyle BDSM types walking into the firing range of bullwhips and quirts. An 18-foot bullwhip has got to have a space at least twice that distance in order for it to swing efficiently. I saw a lot of accidents and so I ended up writing the club etiquette which helped generate enough space for players to avoid unnecessary injuries.

PERMISSION TO SPEAK: Captain Zip

Captain Zip has been a part of the fetish scene since the mid 1970s. A talented writer and performer, he writes about his passion for the London Fetish Scene website. He has also compered events at Kinkfest.

'I've been interested in the fetish scene for thirty years. You have to remember that it was the fetish scene that inspired punk and not the other way around. Punk then pushed fetish in a new direction.

'I sent off for some rubberware that I saw in an advert when I was in my mid-twenties. I liked to dress up. I had my first gas mask when I was eighteen. Fetish was something that I had been waiting for, I suppose. My father was a Beefeater, which might explain my passion for tights.

'I have quite a broad interest in the fetish scene. People assume I'm gay, when I'm wearing my nun's outfit, for example, but I'm not. I was on a TV programme once called Secret Suburbia *and I thought I'd come in for a lot of stick from the people who live nearby. But I had quite a lot of people thanking me for helping them. That said, there's still a lot of intolerance out there.*

'I've noticed over the years how the fetish scene enjoys phases. One month there'll be a lot of sad, badly dressed trannies at the fetish market, or a preponderance of latex wearers, and the next month there'll be a lot of hard-looking gays. It's an extraordinary mix.'

One day I was doing the Club Wicked Christmas Party. I had a table full of slaves: Benson, Mouse, Master Don and his slave girl, German Karl-Heinz, a film producer over for holiday ... there were about twenty of us on this large dining table and it was difficult to communicate with them all, so I asked the General – who owns the club – for some bondage rope. All the slaves were wearing collars so I tied them up and pulled on the rope when I wanted to talk to them. A nice idea, I think. At the end I was handing out promotional stuff of mine, free CDs and photos, and Mistress Alexia came over and said she really appreciated what I was doing with the etiquette side of things, making things safer, actually getting off my arse and trying to do something. A lot of people want this etiquette, but when someone does it, it gets criticised, or they believe they're the author's rules, and not a general guide to safety. But that's not the case. I'm just informing people of a good, basic set of rules to ensure safe playing. If my ideas aren't spot on, someone can always come along and finesse them. They're just guidelines. Most clubs have rules and all have security staff and dungeon monitors because the fetish scene now is getting so drug orientated that things can get out of hand and somebody could get hurt. The thing about BDSM is that you really need to be sober and in control in order to do it correctly and safely.

I was asked to look after new upcoming mistresses in clubs so I thought it would be a good idea to tutor them. So I tutored them freely on site and as time went on and I became more popular I had women coming up to me and asking to teach them skills. I started charging between £30 and £50 an hour depending on their budget and my financial needs. I'm not really endangering my own position as a Domme or encouraging competition because there's already a lot of competition out there. There are about 180 Dommes in London alone. Renting a dungeon is £50 per hour. Dungeon masters might end up becoming unstuck if a number of us decide to club together and rent a bigger place for less money in order to do our work. It remains to be seen as to whether that will happen.

When it comes to tuition, I don't really look for pupils, they come to me. I've inspired lots of women to follow in my footsteps. The women will watch me at a stage show because they are trying to learn the trick of how to twist men. It's as if I put them in invisible twine.

For example, Captain Clit approached me at a House of

Flesh party, which was part of the Skin 2 Rubber Ball weekend. It's a place where lots of posers dressed in rubber go to be peacocks for the evening. All the women have got size 8 figures and the men are body builders. Playing-wise it's not that great. I usually avoid them because there's a lot of show ponies and grandstanding. I don't really want to put on a rubber frock and strike poses all night. I'd rather put on some leather and crack some arses.

Captain Clit had seen the TV show and asked me to train her. I gave her my phone number, told her what my fee was and we went from there. After seeing the Captain under my tutelage I can say she's got some talent. But I can't see her having the ability to be a superior mistress because she hasn't got the patience. You have to be a carer as well as a punisher. She doesn't have a very tactile side to her. She told me she hasn't got time for everything I do in session. She wants to punish someone and that's the end of it. And good luck to her.

A lot of the younger trainees respect me and wouldn't infringe on my territory anyway, thanks to the filming I've done, and the reputation I've built up. But I don't think they really have it in them to compete with me, anyway. I haven't seen any really young girls with any great skill. A lot of the best Dommes are in their forties and fifties. It would be quite rare to find a quality Domme between the ages of 24 and 34. Most of the younger ones come from modelling, porn or they've started out as submissives, been trained by masters and then gone off on their own, which pisses the masters off. I'm about the only one – apart from being trained with the quirt under Master Alex – who hasn't really served anybody in a true sense. I'm the only one who has come the other route: sexual explorer turned Domme, rather than submissive turned Domme. Being a sub first gives you valuable experience and I've made sure that I explore that side of things too. But most of the others are in it for the money. If you can make between £80 and £150 per hour alongside a full-time job it's a nice little earner. I try to think of the bigger picture, though.

The first lessons with pupils are about getting back to basics. I have so many different skills but it's important to learn the most common things first. How to cane and flog properly, what gloves to wear, what outfits. General advice will be dispensed regarding what to wear depending on different scenarios. The way to speak to a slave, how to inject your voice with gravitas, that's an important feather to have in your cap too. Being able to dominate a slave with words alone and understanding the benefits of trigger words so that you can read these people without them having to say anything to you is a great skill to have.

You don't need to be the best-looking woman in the world; it's better if you have the capacity for mental play, plenty of lip, knowledge of how to trip people up by simply talking to them. And knowing when to stay silent. Little tricks like knowing to wipe the cane down before and after a caning, especially if the skin has been broken and there is bleeding. And to wipe the slave down too, asking how he is, reassuring him. How the heel of a boot should be cupped. The different positions that a slave should adopt within the dungeon depending on what is happening at any given time. How to kneel and obey, kowtow, that sort of thing. How to choreograph the entrance of a slave and where the mistress would best be positioned when that happens. It's also good to point out that it's best not to drink in session as it can impair your judgment. It's all about basics, simplicity, common sense.

The slaves I choose to be guinea pigs in sessions with trainees don't have a choice ... but most of them are all too happy to offer themselves as experiments. Usually I'll get Rooster or Daphne or Twin to stand in during a training session because they know what to expect. I'll get them together and tell them what they have to do. They're okay with it because they trust my judgment and know that if there is any hard caning to be done it will be me doing it. I wouldn't allow a novice to wield a cane full tilt under instruction. Until they've maintained some kind of accuracy, that is. So the way you get them to improve their accuracy is by getting some lipstick and you draw a horizontal line across the slave's bottom, where the bottom joins the base of their spine, and a line just below the buttocks – it's about a six-inch wide zone. Nine times out of ten they'll do it okay, but occasionally they'll come out of that line. So you tell them it's better to come lower than higher, because the kidneys can be damaged, whereas the tops of the thighs, although painful, aren't going to sustain any long-lasting injury. You also point out that lower on the bottom might provoke an erection in men. Not all do, but around ninety per cent experience this. If you can get the marks of the cane within a half-inch gap you're doing well, a quarter-inch and it's exceptional. I think I can get it under that ... but then I've caned over 5000 bottoms in my time.

PERMISSION TO SPEAK: Slave Rooster

'I've tried other mistresses under Spider's supervision, at parties and clubs, but I didn't like it. I found it too brutal. There was one mistress who gave me a whack in the balls before we'd even started. I used my safe word and she couldn't believe how I'd caved in straight away. But there was no build-up. No sense of her knowing me or my limits before we settled into the session.

'I'm not after a beating. I might like being beaten, but there's a subtle difference. My pain threshold has changed a little, but essentially I'm still the same. It's all about the mental state. The difference is that my sessions occur on the spur of the moment. I don't really book ahead. So I have to get into that zone almost immediately, unlike most slaves who might have three or four weeks before their appointment, time in which they can reach a state of preparedness where they're ready to accept pain. I can't take as much as I think I can because of this. But it's the way I prefer to do it.'

Other safety lessons include no flogging around the face, no electrics above the waist because of the heart, you just have to be aware of basic anatomy and the slave's own needs. If you're too rough with them, they never come back, and you have to remember it's a business, it's what you need. You also have to be aware because it could be the press coming to see you and try to get you in a honey trap. There'll come a time when trainees no longer need my services. But there's some things that only an experienced mistress can teach, such as piercing cocks with needles.

The quirt is my weapon of choice and I practise a lot. I try to get that across to potential dominatrices. Practice is important, even for the best. And you should know your weapon inside out, which is why I will use it on myself. I practise two or three times a week. It's nice. When I practise I'll occasionally whip myself around the back of my bum and legs or the middle of my back, it's a wonderful experience, a nice sting. Twin is being tutored with the quirt but hasn't been able to cut me with it yet, and it's important he learns to do that because I need that peculiar kind of pain.

I don't teach pupils my sensual tricks when I'm tutoring. Or how to have a different style from everyone else. That kind of thing can only come from within you. You have to develop your own voice. It's impossible to teach. And it wouldn't work to have Spider clones everywhere anyway. You have to have your own style, imprint your own quirks, derive your own authority.

One of the nicest tutoring sessions I supervised was when I introduced the Captain to waxing with Clingfilm. She couldn't understand what the benefits were of wrapping someone in Clingfilm. I think there is some kind of odd reaction when you pour various hot and cold liquids on top of it. I got her to wrap Daphne up and we spattered his arms and armpits with molten wax. I've spent lots of time exploring sexually with men and women, so I have a good clue where all the erogenous zones are. Trying different things in those locations can result in some powerful sensations. Another good trick is to put ice under the Clingfilm so when they move they get cold water trickling into different areas of their body. Visually it looks very nice too. If you hook their balls up to a pulley and tug on them while the ice and wax is winding around their flesh it can be quite amazing.

All the time you're explaining the reasons why you're doing this. And it's a good idea to keep in mind that, although you might order a slave to tidy up the dungeon after the session, you must then go around afterwards and make sure everything is absolutely spick and span. You can't rely on these people to do a good job. They might be a bit slipshod on purpose because they want to be punished, but it's crucial the dungeon is in good shape for the next client. You don't want him to find someone else's come in the dog bowl, or blood on the pinwheel that he wants run over his balls. If that does happen, you can expect your clients to not stick around much longer.

PERMISSION TO SPEAK: Captain Clit

'I arrived in the UK two years ago from Hong Kong. If I had pursued my interest in BDSM over there, or anywhere in Asia, I would have been regarded as sick in the head.

'I saw Princess Spider on TV. At a party I asked her if she would consider training me. She is a nice warm person, a good mistress, a good mother. She works hard and she's a good teacher too.

'I'm quite open-minded. I want to follow Spider, but develop my own skills. I want to experiment. I like the power that comes from being in control of a person. I feel safe. Because of some unpleasantness that happened to me when I was a child, I have a fear of emotional and physical hurt. It is through BDSM that I feel I can regain control, and get rid of my demons for good.

'You have to have an interest in others, a real curiosity about people and what makes them tick. I could talk to people I meet for hours. The way they talk, or sit, the things they say and *how they convey their feelings, it is all extremely fascinating to me.*

   '*I am not a hard player, like Princess Spider. I like the sensual side. A lot of people prefer soft play. Not everyone can, or wants to play hard. I like to gently tie up my clients and leave them feeling helpless, but not to fear anything that might be about to happen. I like to play games mentally with them. Arouse them, make them feel that they can have me sexually, but never allow it. Even the most experienced slaves want to try something new.*

   '*I would like to explore this side of things more. I like the idea of mental challenges, of taking different ideas from different people and throwing them into the mix, see if I can come up with new ways of stimulating people. You begin to understand people more and it helps you to compare yourself with them. I find it a handy psychological tool. It helps me to improve as a person.*'

Most people think they can buy a crop and become a mistress, but you need someone who knows something about it to tutor you. The first time I went to a fetish club with Simone back in my early London days I met this guy who is a good friend of mine now, Master Alex. He makes his own whips and he loves girls. He thought I was submissive and he wanted to spank me. He asked if he could spank me and I said, 'Yes, you can play with me, but I'm interested in your whip.'

   He had a long bullwhip and it was too long for me, I've never been very strong, and asked if he had anything shorter that I could try. He desperately wanted to play with me and he gave me this quirt, which is my specialised weapon. I was just standing there and he was showing me how to use it. You can put something on the end, a cracker, a little tail, to make it crack like a bullwhip. I said I wanted one. But he started me off with a flogger, which is short, with a handle, and lots of tails, sometimes soft, used to warm people up before moving on to the heavy duty equipment. I got him to show me this quirt and I just flicked the tail and he bent over a bench and the idea is to get it on a certain area of the backside because it can stimulate an erection and he said you can go a bit harder. And he said: 'You're a natural. You're the first person I've met who knows how to use this thing properly.'

So I took the flogger and started playing around. There was music, and I like to move around, so I was moving to this music, playing with this flogger, and I looked around and there were all these blokes lined up waiting for me.

Alex was my tutor where weapons are concerned. He actually lent me the flogger to do this big guy. I made him look puny with this amazing weapon. Alex loved it and we became great mates. He was my entrance into getting the skills.

You can have a mistress persona and not be a mistress, and you can have a lifestyle mistress and not want to be a pro-Domme. You have to have something about you that the blokes find dominant, maybe the boots you wear, whatever. You don't really have to have a dungeon. It doesn't make a difference where you are.

The next person I met after Alex was at SM Pride which has now become the annual event known as KinkFest and I was with Graham and went in a black velvet dress and this man of about fifty in a schoolboy's uniform came up to me and said, 'Miss, would you cane me?' and I looked at Graham because Graham doesn't like the cane so he hadn't showed me how to use it. And Alex at that time hadn't taught me how to use it, so I thought to myself, how am I going to get out of this? But I said, yeah, okay, select your weapon.

A woman came over to me and said, 'He likes quite a hard caning, would you like some instruction?' I said, yes, that would be nice, and she was Miss Prim, who actually runs a whole school, The Muir Academy, in Hereford where adults go to be schoolboys and schoolgirls. I didn't know how big she was in the BDSM scene until later.

She showed me where to aim and I used to play tennis so I thought I'd give it a go as if I was executing a powerful forehand smash. I focused on the target, made sure the tip landed on the flesh and WHACK! She said I was a natural, so suddenly there were a few things I was good at and I thought, right, stick to those for the time being.

That guy, my first ever cane victim, still comes up to me in clubs and wants me to give him six of the best. It was a case of right place, right time. I learned from Miss Prim all about the school scenes, which I really got into. I quite like to play a prefect role, not old enough to be a teacher, so I can be a bit mischievous, grass people up and get them into trouble or help the teacher in class with punishments, after all, the pupils are there because they want to be caned ...

The way it goes in the mistress world, the old dears who are now in their fifties are being replaced by a younger breed who just don't have the same kind of personality and presence. I used to wonder about how I could spread the word about what I was doing, try to reach a wider audience. I knew there were slave boys of forty to sixty years old visiting the mistresses who are now retiring and didn't have any time for the new wave of harder, less traditional Dommes. They were people I could work with because I have embraced those old-style methods. I talked to some of them and realised they were a dwindling customer base. They weren't being catered for any more and so they were turning away from the BDSM world.

I started a campaign. I used to make up ten CDs of stories and pictures and give them to various guests at parties. It was a big expense but it was media flooding and it was worth it. I didn't want to be one of the 'Spank and Wank' brigade. I was determined to follow the training routines of the older ladies. An eastern European mistress shook my hand once and told me she had the utmost respect for me, that I was doing fabulous stuff. She liked the little things, the way I never lit my own cigarettes, that people in my company were to always keep their heads at a lower level to mine. Very basic courtesies.

There are lots of ritualistic things like that that have been passed down so I train my ladies in the way that I have learned. I teach them how to use the equipment and the safe words, I tell them what the slaves are feeling. A lot of mistresses can't or won't switch, so they don't have any empathy. I went to a party called the Bossy Brigade and there was Mistress Alcala, Wolf, Culleen, Scylla, myself and others. The theme of the party was forced bisexuality. We had a pre-party meeting to talk about how the night might go and I asked if any of them had ever switched. They looked at me as if I'd asked them, 'Do you speak Martian?' Well of course they hadn't.

I asked them how could they possibly know what it feels like to be caned? And they just said that they didn't know. They caned them without that knowledge. The same where needles were concerned. None of them had ever had a needle inserted through a nipple. They didn't understand that there were different flavours of pain that existed. I felt there was an essential element missing in their lives. So many out there don't switch. I think it is possibly the most important thing a mistress can do, experience the life of a sub. Once you know how it feels, you know how to give it.

Introductory letter from Mistress Juan (couple scenario):

My slave has been instructed to introduce himself and request an audience with you for instruction and correction, with a view to teaching him how to treat goddesses such as ourselves. Since I find him at times wayward and disobedient, and at best uncommunicative and slow to respond, I feel I need some help to teach him how to behave. I have noted with interest your TV work and like your attitude, which reflects my own desire to be cruel but caring. To chastise is good, to damage is not my goal.

My slave has only one physical problem area which is a weakness of the back (not to be confused with being spineless, which, of course, they all are). Other than that he appears strong and with whips, canes, lashes, hairbrushes, etc. has managed to cope with a fair number of strokes (500 mild, 50 hard).

He enjoys dressing up in feminine garb and is used to humiliation. I frequently send him out, or even escort him, while he wears feminine underwear beneath his clothing. I do not send him out with feminine outer clothing as he is most unconvincing. This is solely so I am not humiliated by association, you understand.

I look forward to our meeting, and thank you for agreeing to accept him as a supplicant, and myself as a trainee mistress.

We put the slave on his knees and I'll ask Mistress Juan what she does with him and what he likes. The last session we had he wanted to be a maid. He had brought along some fabulous red tights – I really wouldn't have minded a pair myself – and we put him in some high-heel shoes. He's also wearing a wig. He's stumbling around. He's quite tall with an angular jaw and square shoulders. The picture doesn't fit. There's potential but something isn't quite right. I'm asking her what she thinks of his tottering, and I say to him, 'You have to totter if you want to be a maid.' So I got Mistress Juan to show him how to totter. I said, 'Would you like to see Mistress totter?' and just changed my voice a fraction, made it softer, made it warmer, and I know what they like, so I showed him: 'Look, you have to wiggle your bum, you have to walk on the balls of your feet. Prowl.'

And he thinks he's got it. And it's far too easy, so I tell him I have to go and get something and I nip off to find a tray. And I load it with glasses of water and he's now got to walk with this tray, curtsey, and he's six foot something and he's got to get down to curtsey and suddenly it's not so easy any more. And he spills a bit and there's an excuse to stop all the tottering nonsense and get him over a bench and cane him.

He wanted anal play and he said he was ready and I was just about to do him and he said, 'Mistress, I haven't emptied my bladder,' and so I said, 'Silly girl,' and sent him off to the toilet with his tights around his ankles, tottering away, a real sight. He came back and I lubed up his hole and I was about to stick this butt plug in when I had a thought and I said, 'Have you fasted since yesterday?' as he is supposed to.

'No, Mistress.'

'Well then this is going to be very difficult, painful and messy.'

And Mistress Juan is picking up on my behaviour, the nuances of it, getting the hang of it now, saying, 'Mistress, this is unacceptable.' She's understanding the attitude you need, the edge to your voice, the menace. I'm not really tutoring her as much as giving her encouragement to show her true colours. We're ganging up on him and she's feeding off that.

We try to get this butt plug in, the smallest bugger in the dungeon, and it just won't go in. So more lube. And it's the noises that are important, she can see that now. The squelch of lube, the thwack of a latex surgical glove on a buttock; he's blindfolded and twitching with every tiny sound. She's learning by being in the thick of it. I showed her the butt plug has a rubber stopper to prevent it getting lost inside and you just use the flat of your hand and press until it's flush. And it's going in at last and I say to her, 'Would you like to fuck your slave?'

And she's obviously been waiting for this for a long time and she pushed it in quite hard and he yelped so you have to show her that the anatomy isn't exactly straight, there are curves in there and you have to be gentle and coax it in different directions. He found it quite enjoyable even though he hadn't fasted and we ended up having to clean him and chastising him for being so messy and decided that a suitable punishment for him would be to pole dance for us in his high heels. He had to dance erotically for us. You never saw a grown man so humiliated in his maid's outfit, lop-sided wig, high heels and tights. He was gyrating like someone pissed or injured and Mistress Juan was choked up with laughter. She said that not many women would come up with so much inventive stuff.

She told me he wanted to masturbate over my feet. I said, 'How long has he been in training?' She told me, not that that was important, but it was all a way of teasing him, and I said,

'That sounds reasonable. But I'm taking my stockings off, I don't want him ruining my stockings, these were £18 a pair.' And now I roll my stockings off and offer my feet to him and say, 'How lucky you are, slave, to have Mistress's naked feet, look at my little painted toenails ...' and he's got an erection of course, how could he not with these beautiful little feet all his to play over?

He's perspiring, his lipstick's smudged, his tights are all over the place and I tell him he'll have to strip. Mistress Juan asks me what I'll be doing while he has a wank and I tell her I'll smoke a cigarette while the maid plays with her pussy. Now I've put him in a female scenario he's in gaga land. So we're both watching him bring himself to orgasm, and I've got my feet positioned before him, giving him a little view up between my legs. And eventually he comes all over my feet – and remember, I wouldn't normally do that for a single paying client, I'd normally let him come over my boots or something – I broke a few rules there but they're so nice I thought, what the hell. And then it was into the medical room with him for a golden shower. We lay him in the wet room and I cocked my leg up and peed all over him. I said, 'Right, I'm going off to get cleaned up. Mistress Juan, it's your turn. Finish him off.'

She laid him out completely flat. She hadn't been to the toilet for over two hours and she drenched him. But the whole point is that you can't work out how to tutor them until you can see a glimpse of how they play at home. With that pair it's light, low-level punishment and lots of erotic sensual stuff with verbal and visual humiliation for him.

Session Review by Slave M:

We were shown down to a changing area where I was to dress in a maid's outfit and as instructed in a previous email from Princess Spider I had to put on some bright red tights. I assisted Mistress Juan to change into her blue corset, stockings and new shoes. I then followed my Goddess into the dungeon where the evening's events would take place.

The dungeon was a lot larger than the previous one we had attended. There was a feeling of space yet a sense of confinement. There were numerous items around the room which I could be tied to or punished over. The lighting was subtle but bright enough to be able to admire the beauty of both mistresses.

Soon I was ordered to kneel on the floor in front of Princess Spider's throne. Princess Spider made me clean her black boots with my tongue; she said they had been made dirty and dusty from her trip to the dungeon on the train. I set to work licking the leather all over making sure every speck of dust was removed. After a while Princess Spider vacated the throne and Mistress Juan sat there so I could worship her shoes, followed by her feet.

Later Princess Spider again sat in the throne and I had to read out passages from my homework book to amuse the mistresses. Various emails contained homework for me to do prior to this visit. After that I had to worship Princess Spider by kissing and licking her feet after she had removed her boots, this was followed by kissing all the way up the legs to her stocking tops. As a slave I was not allowed to go any higher or I might get punished.

I had been given a tray with drinks on it to hold for my mistress, this I had to carry around the room without spilling any drink. The task was difficult, as I was not used to walking on a polished floor with high heels. I suppose I should practise more in the shoes. Every now and then I had to walk up to one of the mistresses and curtsey, as every maid should be able to do. A spanking followed this task across a bench, which I had been instructed to place in the middle of the room. Further deportment training took place before I was sent to clean the floor at the far end of the dungeon. I was soon back on my knees going around the floor with a dustpan and brush, trying not to miss any dirt in case I was further punished.

During the session I had to massage Princess Spider's legs and feet with some massage cream we had brought along as a gift. This was a pleasant treat to be allowed to do. I had carried out this task many times in the past on Mistress Juan.

In the centre of the room was a metal pole going from the floor to the ceiling. I was to entertain both mistresses by giving a display of pole dancing. I tried but my abilities in this field were not very good. I soon found myself being tied to a piece of the dungeon furniture in a kneeling position with my rear exposed. Princess Spider was going to instruct Mistress Juan on how to dominate me with a strap-on. The first part was to relax me and this was done by a spanking, followed by a hard caning. Mistress Juan and Princess Spider carried this out in turn and sometimes together. I had been blindfolded and Princess Spider had removed her knickers and placed them in my mouth, much to the delight of Mistress Juan. The punishment was hard and I still have the marks to prove it over a week later. Mistress Juan had the opportunity to try out various implements to strike me with. The lesson with the strap-on followed.

After the strap-on lesson I was stripped in front of both mistresses. Princess Spider then lay down on the floor and I had to kneel by her feet. I was then instructed to rub myself over her feet and give myself relief while being encouraged by Mistress Juan. Eventually I came all over Princess Spider's feet and toes and guess who had to clean them up?

The session was drawing to a close but Princess Spider decided I needed to be taught a lesson and in the shower room it was my turn to be down on the floor. Princess Spider stood over the top of me and I was given a golden shower, which lasted what seemed forever. I was left to clean myself up before getting dressed.

This was a good session for Mistress Juan and me and I hope Princess Spider enjoyed it as well. We look forward to more encounters in the future. Hopefully the cane marks will have gone by then.

I also have a lovely couple who come over to see me from Ireland on a regular basis. She's another one who enjoys me tutoring her in the domination of her partner. Lucy first saw me in the *Mistress Files* magazine. She waited for two years to see me. Her schedule and mine just wouldn't allow it. We finally met in Club Wicked. She came to me and gave me a big kiss. It wasn't until she opened her mouth and spoke to me and I heard her Irish accent that I realised who she was. Everyone thought she was my lost girlfriend.

She wanted me to punish her lover. She had the money right there. I took her outside so she could pay me and then went back in and caned him. Otherwise it would have been a serious breaking of etiquette. You're not supposed to take payment in clubs, it's like prostitution. Inside I got John up on the cross and spanked his arse and then quirted him. Lucy interrupted me, not realising that you should never do so during a session, it's absolutely forbidden. Already she had demonstrated that she needed some good guidance from a teacher. She told me that perhaps I ought to take it a bit easier. I was taken aback because she had told me he liked it hard. 'Yes,' she said, 'but I didn't realise you could cane like that.'

They're a nice couple. I like them so much that it doesn't matter to me that they break rules and drink in session. They always bring booze and have a couple of glasses. I will limit myself to just one. Lucy will sometimes play as a mistress alongside me and we'll both dominate John. He likes caning, pussy-worship, bottom-worship, humiliation. He's got a great big dong and we always tell him it's the smallest thing we've ever seen. He's something in politics or diplomacy and they are always travelling all over the world. They give me fabulous gifts and lots of money when they come to see me. They're very generous. The last time I saw them I got a thousand pounds for two sessions over two days. The dungeon fee was £150 and so I was seriously in pocket afterwards. They've bought me some great leather boots in the past. I see them once every two or three months.

They're good because I'll get a call from Lucy saying, 'Can you set up a game?' And I'll say yes, where? 'Anywhere. It doesn't matter. We'll be there.' Whatever I set up, they've never been disappointed. I'll set up a dungeon and a time and a scenario. Lucy always wants to know what the game is. I never tell her.

It's a bit more informal when we're in session. We'll swear at each other and joke and call each other by our first names. It's all a bit of a giggle. They can do anything, they're happy with any kind of session. They are my favourite couple. She wants to learn how to do things. She's quite a fan of mine. I'll get a call from them from some far-flung location, and they're playing. 'I've got this naughty boy here,' she'll say to me. 'What should I do to him?'

'Spit on him!' I'll say, and I'll put the phone down.

Or recently I got a call and she said: 'He's here with me, the man.'

'Oh yes? Has he got an erection?'

'Yes. He wants to know what the game is.'

'Tell him the game is snooker. I'll see you Friday.' And I'll put the phone down. It's very playful.

From *The Feminisation of Daphne*

My name once upon a time was Peter. I had all my life thought of myself as a normal male of the species even during my life as a slave, albeit a lowly one. I had all the normal feelings that most men have concerning their sexuality. Then in July 2003 I entered into a slave contract and became the property of Princess Spider. I was given the slave named Daphne. At the time I was thinking that being given that name was a form of humiliation and I thought little more of it. As the months followed it never dawned on me that out of all the slaves that belong to my Princess, I was the only one who had been given a girl's name.

Time went by and the ownership that my Princess had had became complete and her control over me was total. My sex life had diminished by this time although I did used to masturbate reasonably often and when I came it was caught in a tissue and disposed of. It was the normal thing to do.

That was until October of this year when this practice changed abruptly. This time I had caught my cream in my hand and without thinking about it I had swallowed it. Why I did this I do not know but it seemed such a natural thing to do.

Then came the day that was to turn my life upside down. A few days prior to being taken to a multi-mistress party I had been instructed to buy some hold-up stockings and a mini-skirt. A couple of days before the party I had obtained a butt plug and started using it on myself. This seemed so natural, but the penny still hadn't dropped.

The night of the party arrived and I was instructed to change and felt so comfortable wearing my stockings and skirt in front of others. I was taken into a room and told to lie over a bench, my skirt was pulled up, I was told to spread my legs. I felt myself being lubricated and then my Princess entered me with a strap-on she had slipped into. Another slave was brought to the head of the bench and I was told to start sucking his cock. I found myself doing this not because I had to but because I wanted to. When my Princess had finished another mistress took over with a longer dildo and I had to suck more cock. A lot of it. It was ecstasy. Then the bombshell hit me. What I was enjoying so thoroughly wasn't due to any bi or gay tendencies, it was due to Daphne. I suddenly realised that Daphne had been there all the time and that my Princess had brought her to life. My Princess must have sensed that I had this exceptionally strong feminine side within me and now was the time for it to come to the surface. Later on that evening I found that as Daphne I begged my Princess to take me again. I begged as a female slave.

The days passed and I was soon wearing suspender belts, stockings and panties on a full-time basis and my mini-skirt when indoors. My butt plug is used on a daily basis for four hours at a time and I use suction cups on my nipples for several periods each and every day in the hope they will become permanently enlarged. I also bought a ring for my wedding finger to show that I'm owned. I now keep my body totally shaved at all times.

A lot of this feminine transformation has taken place in my mind and I now find myself thinking only as Daphne. I still milk myself because I love the taste of it but don't do it as often as before. I find myself playing with my nipples more often and fingering the G-spot behind my balls. A larger butt plug and dildo are on my shopping list to use in what I now call my 'pussy arse'. I also have a longing to pleasure and satisfy men as they use me as the whore in Daphne emerges.

The mental feminisation is now in a short space of time complete. Peter no longer exists. What does truly exist and is here to stay is the true and feminine slave Daphne. In addition to being known only as Daphne I do have a wish and that is that no matter whose presence I am in I am thought of and referred to as a 'she' and not a 'he' and as a 'her' and not a 'him'.

The physical side of this transformation has just begun. Yet to come is obviously my wardrobe so that it has a good range of feminine clothes, tuition in the proper use of make-up, training in deportment when wearing high heels, wigs or a feminine hairstyle, voice training and, if it can be obtained, hormone therapy.

I will always be a total punishment and torture slave to my Princess but I no longer serve in that role as a male slave. I can now only truly serve my Princess as her true female slave Daphne.

There is one final thing that must come under the realm of training. My Princess, over the months, you have always given me a free rein in my role as your slave. I have come to feel that maybe subconsciously I have not been 100 per cent in serving you.

Maybe because of all the freedom, I feel that at times I may have become a bit complacent, resulting in not always putting all of your interests before my own. Perhaps it may be time for those reins to be tightly drawn in so that the new Daphne is fully aware of the meaning of the power of the endless total domination and control that you must have over her in all aspects, especially her mind, and that I must serve you not just totally, but totally and more and then more again.

Your devoted slave.

Daphne

CHAPTER EIGHT: SPIDER BITES

'Everyone thinks a mistress needs to be a size 8 or 10, pert breasts, cute little bum ... but it's crap because most guys, believe me, like a much curvier woman.'

Princess Spider

London is playing host to a number of mistresses who really don't deserve that title. Of the 180 in the capital, I'd say that there are maybe twenty in my league. The rest are ladies of the night, or amateurs, or women being driven by partners looking to make fast money. The clever thing about Princess Spider is that because I'm not Mistress so-and-so, I'm not like all the rest. I've got a name that sticks out. I have an image and a logo.

When I decided to call myself Princess Spider, there were suddenly a lot of spider-related items in the zeitgeist. It seemed pre-ordained. When a spider appears on television, I know it will trigger my slaves to think about me. You have to keep thinking of little tricks like that to get into their minds because the BDSM scene is currently at threat from the club side of things. Generally things are slowing down for us Dommes. Slaves just aren't going to see mistresses at the moment. And the mistresses are retiring all the time. Twelve called it a day last year. I think it's down to the growth of fetish clubs. I think it's gradually dying out, I certainly get that impression from other mistresses I've talked to. It's disappearing because of the cane being banned in schools, the lack of parental discipline, clothes not being smart or regimented any more. Men want different things now.

In the old days men wanted to be punished and disciplined. They wanted to hand over the power to you. Now, the first thing I get asked by new clients is: 'Is there any body worship involved?' Well no, you have to earn that. It's changed a lot. Younger men want a quick sexual fix and want to be naughty with their mistress. They might want to come in their lunchtime and masturbate while they watch you masturbate. There's no skill involved. You could do that with anyone.

A lot of people have the misconception that we are no different from prostitutes. I contest that, although I have no qualms about using the sexual side of things to promote BDSM. Sex is used to sell all kinds of things, from cars to shampoo, and that seems to be acceptable. So why not BDSM? There is a sexy, alluring, seductive, often erotic side to it which I suppose would disappear to some extent if BDSM were to ever surface from the underground and become respectable. It's sexy to be mysterious, unknown, anonymous.

PERMISSION TO SPEAK: Captain Zip

'I've played with a lot of mistresses over the years, both dommeing and subbing. I used to have a cellar but no equipment. Just a few steel rings in the wall. It was quite creepy, quite good in a sparse way.

'I met Princess Spider in 2000 at a TV shoot. There was a dungeon scene and they were asking for volunteers for a sub for her. I put my hand up. She used the flogger on me, on my upper back. It was my first experience of anything like that. She was good fun, very playful, very thoughtful. Some mistresses are only interested in what they want. Princess Spider will watch out for your tolerance levels. And she'll know when you're plateauing.

'After that we kept bumping into each other at clubs and we became friends. You could say that I'm a fan of hers. Our paths have been in tandem for a long time now. We share a similar sense of fun. She's full of surprises. You'll be expecting one thing and then suddenly you've got an ice cube up the bum. There are times when she seems to have eight hands ...'

A pro Domme in the business world is a very small digit in it all. You could put a hundred people in a room and maybe one of them will have paid to see a mistress. People get unusual ideas about mistresses. On the whole it's very mundane and many do it just for the money. I know that some do sexual favours, that's their choice. Some of them were actually ladies of the night and turned to domination. And if someone does provide a sexual favour, you can bet it will be on the slave network pretty quickly. It doesn't help that we wear quite provocative clothes. The Dommes tend to wear black, and a utility belt. That's my uniform, my code of colours.

This talk of sex, it's really something of a grey area. I was on the longlist for Sex Worker of the Year at the Erotic Awards, and I didn't quite know how to take that because I've never really considered myself involved in the sex industry. Maybe I am. We advertise in magazines but we also go into websites that are listed alongside escorts. That doesn't really bother me because I've done the escort side of it – not the sex thing, but dinner and showing people around and going to parties – but it's not the old school who are confused, the 40+ guys. They know what a dominatrix is and what it's all about. It's the younger guys who don't have time to find out about it and they lump us in with the same category as the sex workers. And also it's never been classed as a business. It's always had the reputation of being a bit scuzzy because it's cash in hand, no questions asked, that type of thing.

We get a lot of calls for sex from the younger men who can't seem to differentiate between Dommes and prostitutes and it's a shame because it's not really about that, unless you're lucky enough to be a Body Slave. I think I'll end up filtering out that physical side of things and just enjoying BDSM more in private with my partner as opposed to professionally. We all have a natural lifespan anyway. You can only be popular for so long. I give myself maybe another five years, and then I'll probably revert back to new media. Other mistresses are already doing part-time office jobs because they're not getting the bookings they used to. All the fetish shops, the equipment and clothing sellers, they're struggling to make money too, because once you have your outfits, you don't need to buy any more. There aren't so many loyal slaves around now because the whole market has been flooded with so much choice.

You can get naughty phone texts, pay to view. Internet access to any kind of sexual act you can imagine. Before too long this whole BDSM scene will become an internet-based industry. That's fact. People have less time. Transport is worse. There's less time to travel. Why cause yourself all that stress when you can click on the Web and see your favourite mistress? You can pick up the phone and talk to her. I think the majority will get their kicks from the internet. There are a lot of pay-to-view sites too where you pay around £25 to see all your favourite fantasies, even though you're not experiencing them directly – it gives the pervs that are out there their two or three-minute fix when they can have a wank. Which is why I've thought ahead and constructed my own submission site.

It's around £150 to see a mistress these days. In the old days it used to be £250. It's easy to pay £25 for a month's viewing of a website – you don't physically have to do it. You can be anonymous. Some still crave the play and attention, and I think there will always be the need for private sessions, but there are so many fetish clubs now where you can go cheaply and get whacked by ten famous Dommes. It's good value for money. We do it for publicity but in a way we're killing our own business. I started moving away from doing too many clubs. There are more now than there've ever been but obviously there are some fetishes you can't replicate in the clubs, especially the messy ones like anal play and golden showers. Body Slave stuff.

That said, I've still got new slaves contacting me from old reviews I wrote for *Kane* magazine, which is normally the spanking and school play quarter. It's nice because they usually come to me from more conventional BDSM magazines or my own website, www.princess-spider.com.

Most slaves have an urge, it's a spontaneous thing: they want to see you on that day at that time to fit in with their schedule. Most mistresses can't do that. So they'll float around looking for a mistress they can go to when they want to, not when the mistress can fit them in. So that means a mistress with her own dungeon, not one that she's renting, like me. I have to book them in advance. But unlike most mistresses who get these spur-of-the-moment demands, I do get advance bookings. So people will save to come and see me. But I'd like, ultimately, to run everything from home. And as much as I love doing this, we all have a shelf life and who's to say in five years' time there won't be another Domme as popular as I am? Maybe then it will be time to bow out, at the top of my game.

PERMISSION TO SPEAK: Slave Rooster

'BDSM is still underground but it's more accepted now. From a slave's perspective, if slaves knew how good Princess Spider was they wouldn't hesitate in coming to her. But there's a lot of crap out there. Differentiating is hard unless you experience it. There might be people interested in the scene who go to a mistress and think that's it, in terms of quality. They'll either stick with that one mistress or be put off the scene because they've been disappointed by the session and tar all mistresses with the same brush. There's also a lot of people out there who are interested or curious but don't take that final step.

'Her public appearance is a very important part of the whole picture. She's a big woman, she has real presence. With heels she's not far short of six foot tall. She generates attention

whenever she walks into a room. She's gregarious and friendly, but there's this underlying menace, the power she carries, which of course is essential for any successful dominatrix. She looks as if she means business. And yet she cares greatly for her clients too. She chats with you before a session, to understand your psychology and to work out your health background and fantasies.'

Now I'm closer to the end of my career than the beginning, I spend quite a bit of time thinking about the possible triggers in my childhood that inspired these unconventional life choices. I was the eldest child in my family, so of course I was very bossy. I was very competitive. And I've always been an individual, a bit of a loner, striking out on my own, doing my own thing when everyone else was following a trend. I was bullied at school, which forced me to be independent and strong.

I was tall and gawky, I had snow-white curly hair when I was little. I used to talk to these two boys who were nervous about school, and told them stories to calm them down, away from all the other kids. We had this great fallen oak in the playground and I would sit there with them and invent these fantasy places where we could escape for a while. We used to play tigers and lions. My first boyfriend would crawl all over my body while we were playing.

We had this makeshift tent in our garden. Next to my house there was a public footpath running up to the fields. We'd always be in there playing in the straw. Dad would give us some money and tell us to go and buy a cabbage and we'd go up the field, nick a cabbage and keep the money for sweets. I've always had that cheeky resourceful streak. We used to play army games as well. I had thousands of toy soldiers and built lots of models. I had lots of patience for that kind of thing and I still play war games now. But again, it's very tomboyish. The seeds of my need for control and domination can be traced back to that time and the behaviour that I was displaying.

I was good at school, but there was a lot of jealousy

because my dad used to buy me great gear for sport, which I excelled at. I also excelled at a lot of typically boys' subjects: physics, geography, history ... I don't know why. But then I fell for one of my classmates, this girl called Ivy. Someone found a note from her in my bag and I got a horrendous amount of abuse and bullying after that. My marks fell from As and Bs to Ds and Es. I didn't have any support. I was pretty much, along with Ivy, the only gay girl in the school, and we're talking about the early 1970s, when it was virtually unheard of.

I suppose my first initiation into domination was with a girl called Helen. She was 16, I was 17. She was curvy and her hair fell loosely, sexily, over one eye. It made her seem quite mysterious. We'd only been seeing each other for a little while. She liked to be pinned down, which was quite nice. I was in my punk and skinhead phase and she was curious about my chains and buckles and belts. I spent ages hammering studs into a second-hand belt. I used to get quite erotic with her. Considering we were so young it was quite gentle stuff, tender. I'd take advantage of her, flipping her over on her back, automatically assuming a dominant role although I didn't really know what being dominant meant. She was really nice. On one occasion my friends were coming over and they all thought it was a bad idea that I should be seeing her. I don't know why – she was the best and horniest woman I'd dated. Her skin was very soft, she had freckles, she was quite pretty. We were all going clubbing but she insisted I cuff her up to her dad's sofa. Everyone piled in and she was sitting there with a gag in her mouth looking up at everybody with these soulful brown eyes. It was so funny. They completely freaked. We went off dancing and it was my birthday and she was a bit drunk and she got into some trouble with her parents for being out all night. We had sex. My dad knew what was going on and didn't approve but he turned a blind eye. It ended because I was working in Birmingham and she was just leaving school. I was hungry for more exploring, more experiences. That was my first experience of capturing a girl and handcuffing her. It was something of a launch pad.

When it really got going seriously with role play I was with a girl called Maxine who had soft brown curly hair. Very cute. I was wearing a severe skinhead, a number one cut, which sounds unattractive on a girl but it was really my most successful period of being with women, sometimes having three girls a night, which is no mean feat for a seventeen-year-old! We explored different characters together. She sometimes dressed up in a frilly shirt, drew a moustache on her with her eye pencil and pretended to be the Duke of Monmouth. We played lots of games like that.

We had sex that was very lusty, and swapped between being dominant and submissive, although we didn't realise that's what we were doing at the time. It was interesting. I spent seven years with her but only saw a couple of men in that period. In the end I left her and went out with a woman called Debra. She left her husband and we got a house together. That's when I began to explore dominant roles in sex more fully.

Her husband was a linesman and I got to know them while I was coaching a team of young footballers. After school we'd meet up for coffee at her place, the kind of thing mums do all the time. One day I went to see her and she was wearing a skimpy dressing gown with a lacy white body underneath it. I was sitting there thinking, *God, what am I supposed to do?* I knew what I'd like to have done ... Just before I left I said to her, 'You're lucky to still be wearing that with me around. Anybody else and I'd have gone for it.'

She smiled and said, 'Why didn't you?'

I didn't know that she fancied me until that point. The next time I saw her, her husband was at a meeting. We had a horny smooching and groping session. One day he was away on work, our kids were out with babysitters. We had a lovely meal that she'd cooked and afterwards we were leaning across the table kissing. The plates had yet to be cleared away and she ended up on the table with her knickers off, flashing her beautiful little pussy at me. She asked me to come to her. I thought, I'm not playing games so I dragged her towards me and buried my face between her legs. The plates went all over the place. It was a complete mess, but very passionate.

Over a few months there were a few more dangerous liaisons until things came to a head and she moved out. She had real style. She called me up and wanted to play a game. She would be an estate agent selling a house and I would be the potential purchaser. She was dressed in black high heels, stockings, a short pencil skirt and a fitted '50s style jacket, her boobs were trapped in this lacy bra, they were huge breasts, and her hair was pinned up. She was wearing orangey red lipstick instead of her usual deep red, to further the illusion that she was someone else. She was wearing a luscious perfume called *Eden*. She looked very sophisticated.

I knocked on the door and she opened it very formally and my jaw dropped. She wanted me dressed like a man, so I'd put on some shoes and trousers, a grey granddad shirt with pinstripes. My hair was shaved at the time, with little funky dreadlocks, the start of my dreadlock phase.

Inside I was being shown around all the rooms and I'm saying, yes, very nice, and she's started teasing me, flirting with me, giving me various views as she's leaning over to show me bath taps, that kind of thing. And she's wearing no knickers, her pussy completely shaved.

Upstairs she said to me, 'Would you like to see anything else?'

What could I say? I said, 'I want to see it all.'

'If you want to see it all, you have to get on your knees.' She's the first person to ever make me get on my knees. She crossed her legs in this wicker chair and gave me this glimpse of naked fleshy pussy. I could see she was soaking. She got me interested in this business of lingering, where you've got your dessert right in front of your face but you're not allowed to touch.

She allowed me to kiss her thighs, and then she lifted her legs and crossed them around my shoulders. I heard her high heels click together. She said to me, 'You can have just one kiss.'

I've kept that routine with my partners now. It's one of the horniest things I've ever experienced. So I take my kiss and I'm ordered to tell her pussy that I love it. And that was staggering, having to talk to her pussy. So erotic. It might seem a bit straight now, but at the time it was something else.

After an age she let me have a real taste of her forbidden fruit, so I was tonguing her and it all got very passionate and I ended up splitting her skirt up over her arse and I had her on the bed with her bum in the air and I was sucking and licking at her from behind. She's tearing my trousers off and my shirt. It was fiery stuff, very powerful. Sexually, she's probably the most exciting person I've been with in a lesbian way. The games went on like that and we saw each other for five years. One of the things I liked to do with her was choose her outfits for the works parties she went to. I'd pick out the skimpiest outfits for her to squeeze into. I'd get her to wear a skimpy red thong, which always squirmed up her bald glistening pussy when she walked. It used to really torment her. One time she told me it was a mistake sending me out in that skirt and knickers because she had to walk up a spiral staircase and everyone behind her got a great view . . .

She came back with two guys and a woman. The woman was lovely, Spanish, dark-haired. She wasn't bi at all, but I couldn't work out why these guys were there. I guessed she must have been fucking one or both of them.

They were sitting in the lounge and I asked her to come into the kitchen. I locked the door behind her and ripped her knickers off, then finger-fucked her against the door, really getting it rattling in the frame so they could all hear what was going on. After she came I made her lick my fingers and sent her back into the other room with a warning never to be naughty again. But of course, she was. Who wouldn't be, after that?

She was a horny lady and she was there at the start, when my dominant persona began to take form.

I'm happy to trade off on the ignorant public perception that I'm a deviant if it means I can earn a living, provide for my family and have fun while I'm at it. I've met some of the nicest, most genuine people during my time exploring BDSM and if I had my days again, I wouldn't change a bit of it. There's no danger, as Princess Spider, of being perceived as a passive woman, as much of society would like to see women. My independence is threatening to some men, and to others it's a massive turn-on. I fit the world of BDSM and it fits me. Like a leather glove ...

I've been doing this for a long time now, I suppose. I've seen things in the dungeon, done things in the dungeon, that most people will only read about, dream about (fantasise about?). There are some out there who don't accept, can't accept, that this sort of thing actually goes on. I've spent my time drinking in the experiences, learning all the time – I'm still learning – and trying to sharpen my skills, develop new tricks or try out new fantasies. The only thing that could stop my improvement is a lack of imagination, from me or my clients, but we're a fecund lot in that department. The capacity for play is endless.

So at the end of it all, what is it that makes a good dominatrix? The qualities of a good Domme in my opinion are the ability to listen, and also take in all the information a prospective slave tells or confesses to you. The ability to understand their particular fantasies, and why they have the desire to serve, and what makes their minds tick. You can't always re-create all of their fantasies, but you can incorporate elements of their darkest secrets. This always begs the question, do slaves top from the bottom (use manipulation to control the dominant)? I think an amicable pre-session agreement negates that question.

The life of a modern-day mistress is changing. In my case, in my personal life I maintain my very dominant side. I tend to date men with strong personalities as this gives me a mental sexual satisfaction of conquering them. In my home partners get dragged into my dungeon for a lesson in sensual BDSM play. I get a buzz from being tossed on my back by a dominant man; this will always appeal to me. On a professional basis, the buzz comes from pure control and the knowledge in my mind that I am training men to be slaves of the web. The therapy of a session helps them to release their pent-up tensions of everyday life. To see them happy and content after a session or role-play gives me great satisfaction.

I'm a lifestyle Domme. I really live my obsession. Every day I will wear leather even when just going shopping or visiting my local cinema. As the head of my household my responsibilities are many and varied. I'm not a control freak; I'm just very good at solving people's problems. I feel the ability to listen always helps. Often my slaves will ring or drop in for a coffee and a quick chat. I don't know if this is commonplace, but I enjoy their company. Masters too come round to my house for lunch or dinner and we enjoy great banter and good wine. Invariably this leads to the request to spank me. Well, that's another story.

My social life is quite busy and takes me out of the UK a lot visiting friends. If I'm not dominating slaves, then I will be writing about them, planning conceptual ideas for TV, or dreaming up new dungeon scenarios. I also advise and help masters and mistresses with their ideas. Various people call me every day and no two days are similar.

CHAPTER NINE: OTHER SKINS

'I believe that everyone likes to be dominated at some stage in their lives.'

Princess Spider

PERMISSION TO SPEAK: Slave Rooster

'She has three primary personas that she inhabits in life. Princess Spider, mother and Maria. When we're working together she's a mum, a working woman, the day to day. Maria is a different kettle of fish. I've seen her and been out with her. She's very submissive, but I don't see her often because I'm not very dominant. You know where you are with each of these characters, but what you don't know is when she's going to switch. And I'm not joking, she can switch mid-sentence. It's quite freaky, because you're not ready for it.'

As I've said, I'm a lifestyle Domme. If you want to be with me, better have some stamina because 24/7 I drink in this existence. But even I need some slack, a change from being the big boss from time to time.

So meet Maria, my alter-ego. Where Spider is a tough, no-nonsense leather-clad bitch Goddess, Maria is a soft-spoken, feminine submissive. An ultra-submissive. If I'm playing with

Master Alex in a club, he'll just beat me as Princess Spider so he will never get any sexual contact, it will just be very naughty and horny and visual for anybody watching. Plus you've got a great master spanking or whipping a great mistress – a real meeting of minds and personalities. It's especially good for him because I'm probably his most famous pupil. Now he asks me for advice business-wise. He doesn't know Maria exists.

This woman is a pushover. Tell her to do what you want and she'll do it. She's my off switch. She's my tension release. Maria dresses in soft, pale-coloured dresses and is incredibly tactile. Maria purrs like a pussy cat when you touch her in the right places. Maria is in thrall to men and is as pliable as modelling clay when she's in the right hands. Bend her, shape her, turn her into what you want. She'll take it all, without complaint. Maria is a blow-up doll with a beating heart. Here's some of what she does ...

Maria is only ever revealed to the people I'm closest too: lovers, partners. I was talking to Master Mark at a recent party; Rooster was accompanying me. Mark wanted me to go down to see him to shoot a film, so Rooster asked him who he'd like to come along. Mark said, 'Well, bring Spider.' And Rooster told him he thought it would be far more interesting to bring Maria. And Mark said: 'Who's Maria?'

I said to Rooster, 'Tell him about Maria while I go and get a drink.'

I looked up a little later and saw Mark's face light up and then turn to shock as Rooster regaled him with tales of Maria's behaviour. Twin now doesn't want me to expose Maria to anybody other than him, which is understandable, especially when you realise that in the past she's played with three guys at a time. And that was quite interesting, especially as they were all slaves.

I switched one night while I was being Princess Spider at a club. I was slowly drinking a few vodkas and having a cigarette at the bar, and I felt this change in me, so I told everyone to go away and leave me alone for a while. I was wearing black leather jacket and skirt, black gloves, as usual. Daphne thought there was something wrong with me, but I was transforming. I just need that little time to mellow out, so that Spider can slink back into her lair and allow this ultra-submissive side of me to shine through.

After three or four vodkas I got my things together and said, 'Right, boys, we're going home.'

In the car, Benson and Rooster told Daphne that he was going to play with Maria, and he didn't understand at first, but then he suddenly cottoned on that Maria was me.

When we got home, the boys started to get things ready. One cleaned up the dungeon, one put the heating on because I don't like to play when it's cold. Daphne was rummaging in the freezer.

I went upstairs because I needed a little more chill-out time before the main event, and I select something skimpier from my wardrobe: a bra top and a little skirt and I still had my stockings on, so off came the boots and on went a pretty pair of high heels. This is the kind of thing that Maria wears, feminine, non-aggressive.

Rooster came to check up on me and then when I went downstairs they put a blindfold on me, which I prefer, because I don't really like to see who's punishing me. Some people like to look their tormentor in the eye. But that doesn't do anything for me, because it's who's in my mind at that moment who is dominating me, which could be anybody. It gives the whole thing a bit more of an edge for me.

Benson was in charge, playing Master for the evening. They basically tossed me over this bench and one of them started smacking my bottom. Next thing I know I feel this really cold fluid on my bum and my pants are being ripped off but I didn't know who was doing what or what the cold stuff was until later when I discovered it was chocolate ice cream – my best bloody chocolate ice cream they were wasting on my bum! – and somebody was licking it off. After that I was ordered to take part in cock identification. I had to feel a cock and guess who it belonged to. Well I knew what they felt like, so it was pretty easy to guess Rooster. I got a smack though, because Maria isn't supposed to know who Rooster is. So I thought I was being clever but I was caught out. This kind of thing always happens to submissives ... you'd think I would know better with my experience! The next one I kept my mouth shut, I was pretty sure it was Daphne, but I didn't say anything. This went on while they fed me wine and asked me questions or to confess to various misdemeanours. I was kept on my toes throughout, but it's difficult to think logically when you're being physically stimulated or abused.

Master Benson would grab me by the hair and make me kiss his boots and crotch. I remember they had me over a spank bench and I heard a buzzing noise and realised it was a vibrator just as it was fed into my arse. And then there was another one in my pussy. And suddenly there was a cock being shoved in my mouth – to this day I have no idea which one of them it was – but the thing is that masters are always more sexual with their slave girls than are mistresses with slave boys, unless they're Body Slaves. Some slave girls like punishment in session if they're paying for it privately, but even then the master would probably have sex with her. So this session was bound to become very sexual.

All these things were going in and out, I didn't know who was doing what, and suddenly someone's fucking me and, because I know his touch, I'm certain it's Rooster. Someone's grabbing my hair and I'm still sucking this cock – but I don't know if it's Benson's cock or Daphne's cock. And now Benson's fucking me and I'm in and out of consciousness, feeling this whip across my back and Daphne's saying, 'Maria, you're a little slut and you need to be punished,' and he's whipping me. He's been in the scene thirty years and so he's picked up some skills, he knows how to use a whip on someone, whereas the other two were just titting around with it. He's getting me where I need it. My bum's getting really warm and I'm relaxing into it, enjoying the feel of the whip. I must have been over the bench for an hour, but it was probably more because in total we played for about six hours. Then I was whipped on the cross and made to do chores and had some nipple torture and at one point I was totally naked but for stockings.

But the most erotic thing I liked was a noose that went around my neck and being hooked up to the ceiling. My legs went, but only for a short while. I thought I was going to drop but I didn't feel in danger because I know Benson, and although we were in the process of splitting up at that time, and I had started to see Rooster – who flipped about the whole noose episode, it really scared him – if he was going to do anything to me, he certainly wasn't going to do it in the middle of a session. There was no antagonism there, they played together all right, but I really enjoyed that part of the evening.

The ultimate, for me, was being quirted. It's what I love most. But the master has to be able to do it properly. I usually end up suggesting they make positional changes, or do it harder. It's very naughty, as a submissive, to be topping from the bottom like that, but it's the only way I can get what I need from the quirt. I wasn't wearing a hood and so I felt justified in ordering Benson around because they're lethal weapons these quirts, and they can do you a lot of damage.

That session was really nice and it was a typical old Maria sort of session. But now it's sexier with Twin.

On this occasion I'd dominated him all night and he had to go to work early because he had a meeting. I woke up feeling horny and I phoned him up and said to him, 'Oh, Master, Maria's feeling naughty, she wants you to come home.'

He texted me – we usually have a lot of text build-up – to say I was bad and a slut, but that he needed to come home anyway at lunchtime in order to pick up some documents for work. In the morning I had a session with Poppy, I was being Nanny Spider. After the session I was feeling really horny – not because of anything to do with Poppy, but from remembering the night before with Twin.

He was telling me he didn't want me to wear any pants so I was wearing a short skirt and a vest top and, at his request, a pair of black mules. And also he demanded that I was not to look at him when he entered the flat.

One o'clock came and he wasn't there so I texted him again to check he was all right and he said he was on his way and he was going to fuck me, but that when he walked through the door he wanted me kneeling on the sofa with my skirt hitched up, facing away from him. I was thinking, well when do I do this? Because I didn't know when he was going to turn up. So I'm kneeling on this sofa with the TV on and I thought, well when the door goes I'll just turn the telly off, I'm not just going to kneel here waiting for him when he could be another half an hour.

When the door goes I quickly switch off the TV and I'm kneeling there and I can hear him come in and I can hear him walking around, picking up stuff, pouring a glass of water, opening some mail, then all of a sudden I hear this scratching noise and the hair on the back of my neck lifts up: it's the scrape of the cane on the floor as he picks it up. He came over to me, caned me eight times, told me I was a slut, smoked a cigarette and then left. And I was absolutely dripping for him. I lay back and begged him to fuck me but he wouldn't. What a bastard. I was so horny.

He texted me to tell me to put some red shoes on and have a wank on the sofa. He told me to go home and he would see me later. And there was I thinking we'd have an hour together at lunch and he took five minutes and went. My arse was really hurting – he must have been randy.

Later he told me it was the most difficult thing he'd done, to cane me, knowing how horny I was, and just leave me there. He had an erection all afternoon. It was lovely, if frustrating.

Rooster came to pick me up a bit later in the day and he saw something had happened. He said, 'What's wrong with you, you look as if you've been rogered.'

And I said, 'No, not rogered, just headfucked.'

She's the flip-side of Princess Spider. Spider likes rules, hates lateness, that sort of thing. She's a real stickler. But Maria will break every rule in the book and try anything and everything. And I've tried most things in my time. But I think Maria has evolved since she's been with Twin. She was different when she was with Benson. She was more into the physical side and sought beatings and quirtings, but I don't know if it's because Twin torments me in a different way but Maria has evolved into a different kind of creature with different needs – we always call it lingering, we leave each other lingering – you could be on the edge of orgasm and he will just leave me. It's the most frustrating place to be, but it's also nice because in between he's tormenting me with wax, or massaging me, or scratching or spanking me. And then he'll come back and get me to the edge again and leave me again.

In everyday life with me, if I'm not looking after this place, or my bloke's place, I've got to be in charge of something, whether it's the company, or the cats or the kids or the slaves. Maria is my way of kicking back and getting some energy. It's really therapeutic. I can play for hours. I went over to see Twin and I wasn't in the mood for it but two hours later I was. He asked me to masturbate so I did and asked him to get the whip and lightly whip me while I did it. But one thing led to another and he forgot to get it. I came but it wasn't the same and he noticed that. He asked me what was wrong and I told him I really wanted him to whip me. He apologised, but it's like you need it, it's an escape from control in the same way he needs to be dominated. It's good for me because if I experience something as Maria, when a slave boy wants the same thing I know exactly how to do it because I know how I felt. From the way they sigh or move about you can tell you've got someone in the right place, and experiencing it yourself first is invaluable in helping you to do that. Some of the best mistresses have to be submissive sometimes.

From Maria's diary:

30th September

I recall this day as the true beginning of my total servitude to my Master. Master has been a long time in my mind and now I have found the true Master, one I will serve and obey. His cruelty I crave for and now I have been dealt my final card. My collar of ownership. My collaring comes as a surprise and now I must kneel, obey and serve my one and true Master.

My crimes are many and my punishment will commence. Kneeling in stockings, leather skirt and leather gloves, no female underwear is allowed. My legs are to be spread wide and my lips parted so my Master may inspect me. My face is pushed to the floor. I may wear perfume and lipstick.

I must choose my punishment instruments before I may commence my total servitude. Master places my collar around my neck and I am forced to suck his penis and lick his leather boots.

My crimes for the day:

Disobedience: 24 x cane

Argument: 24 x spanks

Feistiness: 36 x quirt

Refusing to obey a command: 12 x crop

Twin doesn't like my stockings so much, he likes my legs to be bare. He puts me in red high heels with the Perspex sole and heel and they're four inches high and very strappy. They're very sexy to wear because you walk in a certain way. Your body is rocking, and you're tottering, and your arse is swinging and it's all very horny. His floor is great to walk on because it's completely dangerous, very shiny and polished wood, so I have to be careful, very slow. In a blindfold, wearing very little – how Twin likes it – often in a Moroccan wrap that is tied around me so that the front or the side is gaping, depending on what he wants. He doesn't always blindfold me, but I insist upon it. He likes to see my eyes but I don't like to watch him doing stuff to me. When I want to see him I'll take the blindfold off myself. He will be sitting on the chair and I will come in wearing very red lipstick and pink nail varnish, because I associate red, the colour I usually wear, with being a mistress. It's a very dominant colour. I'll also wear a purple cat collar with stones in it, or maybe Twin will get me to wear his own slave chains, which is a nice romantic touch. I'll kneel down. Most slave girls will have to be told what to do in session, but I know what's expected of me so I'll get down on the floor and kiss his feet. It's quite a height to negotiate because I'm six foot plus in these heels and sometimes he'll have pity and throw a cushion down for me to kneel on. Sometimes if his feet have been in his trainers all day I'll tell him, 'Oh, Master, your feet are very aromatic this evening, how delightful.' And he'll give me a little slap. He'll leave me there and put his feet up while he has a cigarette. He likes me to do nothing while he smokes. Sometimes he'll smoke and masturbate over me while I'm lying there. You don't know what's coming. It's different torments. He might get me off the floor, remove my clothing, and wrap me in red rope. He ties it loose which is good because when he has me crawling around it changes, the rope moves against my flesh and makes new patterns, or gets trapped around my breasts and pulls them in different directions, or slips deep between my thighs and chafes gently against me. It's very erotic. It's nice because you're blindfolded and you'll feel it catch in a place that's a little uncomfortable, and you know how good it must look to your captive audience. The other thing he makes me do is put me in a pair of tights and he'll rip them, so again, when you're crawling, you'll see the skin through the ladders and holes, everything becoming distorted. He'll cut out holes for my nipples to slip through. Everything becomes available little by little.

I called her Maria because that's my middle name, but I have a love of all things Spanish. I want to live there one day. The climate, the food, the music ... it calls to something in me that is simple and romantic. I always said that when I went to Spain I would be Maria, and not go by any other name. Maria is more like an explorer than anything else. She's an excuse to be naughty. But not naughty in a criminal way, naughty sexual.

There's a pretty active BDSM scene over in Spain too. I had a fantastic experience the first time I went over to see one of their dungeons.

The first dungeon I saw in Spain was all down to a TV show I was doing. I just put 'Fetish' and 'Spain' into the internet. *Pain in Spain* came up and it sounded interesting so I contacted them and asked if they'd be interested in being filmed. They invited us over to check their dungeon out. So I went over for a weekend. It's an old Spanish townhouse. No mod cons, no Englishness. All stripped back and plain. It was lovely. They had a lounge on the first floor that led off to the bedrooms, and the bodega, which had been converted into a dungeon. It had a huge door and stone steps leading down. It was very much like a wine cellar but on the left as you go in there was a modern golden champagne box for peeing. Very voyeuristic: the slave puts his head through the bottom and you can sit on it while everybody watches what is going on. Equipment-wise there were chains and whips and locks and manacles but they had some old stuff that looked as if it was from antique shops. Big heavy crosses and black leather thrones. I liked all the nooks and crannies. There were huge stone arches everywhere, curves that really made a contrast with the flat lines of the benches and tables and chairs. It was a really powerful room. There was a caged area with an iron door. You pushed it open and it was a cell/school room. It was intriguing to have that there, with a blackboard. It shouldn't have worked, but it did.

Our dungeons in the UK are very slick. Most of them have carpets on the floor, and radiators, because really they are just normal rooms that have been converted, and not many of them are actually in the basement. Most slaves don't like to have their knees hurt, so you have some kind of carpet, and that means it's crap for high heels because you can't walk properly and there's no evocative sounds as you walk around. It was nice that the floor in Spain was flat and solid, just how it should be as a dungeon. The sound was brilliant in there. There was no decoration, just bare stone walls. It was cool, with a dry cold smell. You got the feeling in your bones that it was the right place; I certainly got goosebumps when I went in there.

They were BDSM lifestylers, the couple who owned it. She used to work in banks and he was ex-police. She started doing some professional Dommeing, but before that they just lived the life, exploring it as a couple.

I found out through them that they were a part of a circle of people, all Brits, all the way from Xavier down to Andalusia on the coast, all of them into the scene. All couples, players. They meet up every other weekend at each other's places and have a fetish party. They had a Yahoo! Group on the internet called *Spain Pain*. They all had fetish parties but this couple was the only one that had a dungeon. Luckily for us we were there at the time a party was going to be on. They were really nice people there. Some from Germany: a big guy called Klaus who ran a ceramics company in La Manga with his wife Sigi; Colin and Jan, he was a builder, she was an ex-machinist looking for work over there; and Babs and Simon. He was an architect and she sold olives at a local market. We all got on quite well. The big question I remember from the party was whether my boobs were real or false, so I had to prove they were real. Then there was a lot of play going on through the dungeon. I ended up playing with Babs. I coaxed her into it, a kind of trigger trap, I was saying, 'It's great to be spanked. Once you get that warm feeling it's really sexy and you start to get turned on. If you're a man you can get an erection. Women tend to get wet and horny.' The girls were enjoying it, and Sigi was sitting there with her mouth open, not quite believing it. Jan I thought was quite prudish for someone trying to be a lifestyle Domme. Anyway, I was egging Babs on, saying she should give it a go, and she agreed. They had this big redwood dining table decked out with great bowls of fruit and candelabra. I got her to bend over the table, and I've got a bit of a reputation for playing tricks. I like to twist and bend the rules. So I went off to the kitchen and scooped up a cube of ice from this large bucket and hid it in my pocket. I was teasing Babs and I lifted her skirt, exposing her buttocks to the audience which caused a few smiles. At the same time I showed everyone in the room that I had some ice in my hand. Babs couldn't see. I tipped everyone the wink. I started spanking Babs, first with my bare hand and then with a glove on. And once she was turned on, writhing against me, I slipped this ice cube into her pussy and followed it in deep with my fingers. She's howling and gyrating against me while I'm delving inside her, trying to find her G-spot. She's really into it, almost clambering onto the table, in danger of spilling the bowls of fruit and the lighted candelabra. Her hair's all wet, and so's mine, thrashing around like a fury of snakes.

Someone has to grab the candelabra before it sets fire to her hair. The table's rocking and the fruit is spilling all over the place. She's in the middle of an orgasm, trying to climb away from me but jamming her hips down against my fingers at the same time. It was really erotic. Everyone was really fired up and ready for anything. It wasn't until after all the excitement had died down that I learned that nothing like that had ever happened at one of their parties. They played, but they didn't play sexually in fetish. They knew of my reputation and that I worked a lot of clubs and did demonstrations, but nothing had prepared them for that little episode. Babs afterwards took me to one side and kissed me and told me she'd never experienced anything like that in her life. And then Klaus got hold of me and asked me to dominate his wife. 'Oh, Princess Spider,' she said, in this thick German accent, 'Very good. Very, very good!'

Later it transpired, maybe a year later, that the whole group is swinging in fetish. When I went back for another party I had the ex-police commissioner giving me pussy worship under instruction while Babs was sucking her bloke's cock. Rooster was there giving me foot massage. I was in control of it lying on the bed being pampered while all this debauchery was going on around me. I'd instruct different people to switch and swap around. I've done that in clubs a lot if there's a private bedroom where you're not on full display having sexual favours, or playing, or whatever you want to call it. It was okay until the commissioner's wife came up and said 'You're not supposed to do that,' and dragged him off, reprimanded him and took him away for a caning.

The nicest thing about that first occasion was that they were all different characters to the people I'd usually meet. At the second party there were a lot of people from the UK who went to Club Wicked so it was the same old faces, but the first time was good, lots of individuals with different backgrounds mixing for the love of the fetish scene. They were all lifestylers, they get slaves from all over Spain going there. But the real reason I liked it was for the dungeon, it was something else.

I put my belt on and walked down those stone steps. Not tiny steps, great big steps that went down and curved around. I felt so powerful, descending. I felt as though I was assuming more and more control and influence with every step I took. That's why I went back to film because it was brilliant for the website. I wore a WPC uniform for the film and the website, a bit cheeky because of the ex-police commissioner. It really knocked him for six. With my dreads tied back I made for quite a convincing policewoman. But I looked the part. Maybe a bit bitchy with my cuffs and truncheon, but it worked for them!

The nearest I came to being in a real honest-to-God dungeon was at Lady Carla's, when we were filming in Barcelona. You wouldn't even know it was there. There's just this row of houses and you go in this gate and walk down some steps and open a door. It's very dark and mysterious and there's a little bar, lots of heraldic stuff, suits of armour. It was odd to walk in and find a bar but it became a club in the evenings for slaves or private parties. There was a grotty-looking area that was full of grey damp funny-smelling tiles, as if you were in a real dungeon, and it must have been naturally a cellar, because it didn't look touched up or worked on in any way. The walls were dripping and grey. High ceilings. Very sparse. You walk through this gate and there's a row of hoods and equipment and a rack and a spanking bench next to a fetter's wheel that you can strap slaves to and spin them. The way it was set up was very spartan. We tend to clutter our dungeons up in the UK so that it's very visually stimulating. Over there, less is more. It's a dungeon equipped with the bare necessities and as such, it really gets your nerves tingling because all you've got to look at is this vast expanse of naked wall. It's like being imprisoned in a real dungeon. Another section contained whipping crosses, all the big bulky pieces of kit. And in the bedroom, obviously for her Body Slaves, was a large iron bed connected to another cold damp empty room. If you were crawling around in there in the dark, you'd imagine you were in a castle keep. It makes you wonder what they think when they come over here. In the UK we have the toughest reputation in the world for BDSM play. But if you went to the Gate dungeon and then went there you'd think the Gate was much softer.

A dungeon, in the end, can be as pretty or as grim as you like. Beyond the visuals, what matters is the skill of the Domme. I can dominate someone in a six-foot space in someone's living room. A dungeon can be anywhere if you want it badly enough.

I watched a session with Lady Carla when I was in Spain. She's not as tactile as I am, she's very firm. I didn't hear her once ask her slave if he was all right, or if he needed water. I think it might have something to do with us in this country being frightened of being busted. So we do everything by the book.

She was dressed to kill in this black rubber catsuit with lacing up the front, and tall boots that were laced into the outfit. She also had some rubber gauntlets and she was all shiny with lube

– it looked fantastic. She has long blonde hair and she was speaking in Spanish.

The session lasted for about an hour. What she did that I liked, and that I'd never seen before, was to get her slave to kneel down while she lit a cigarette. She drew this cigarette gently across his skin, and then her nails, and kept changing things around. It was really sexy because this guy was really hairy. The guy didn't move an inch. And everything just sounded more powerful with that lyrical Spanish voice.

The mistresses in Europe, broadly speaking, look a lot tougher than we do. They spend their money wisely, they have fantastic clothing. For example, there's Mistress Madienne. Her online advert has her in the bath in this black rubber outfit, completely concealed – all you can see are her eyes and her mouth – and she has this elaborate rubber tubing network coming out of and going into this amazing hooded catsuit. They tend to wear things that are weird and menacing. And the slave boys I've talked to about this tend to find it really intriguing, which is half the battle won if you're a Domme looking for a clientele. And also, if you're German and you speak German, you're going to sound menacing, or if you're Spanish and you're shouting, you're going to sound menacing.

On a skill footing, it's different. I've got this couple who have travelled widely, seen a lot of mistresses and, although some of them have been going for 25, 30 years, according to them, I'm a lot better than any of the ones they've seen. I sent them to Maitresse Claudette in Paris a couple of months ago because they were there and on the look-out for a decent Domme. So I put them in touch with her and asked them to let me know how they got on. I got a phone call telling me she was crap and that I was a thousand times better than her. It's all subjective, of course, but I think it's reasonable to say that UK mistresses are more skilled, and harder, than their continental counterparts.

Sometimes I operate as if in a delirium, my identity waxing and waning. I have to work out who I am by what I do.

I once went out as Princess Spider and left Benson in the dungeon, in his hood, cuffed, with a bowl to pee in. His legs were tied but he could move a little. I was wearing a cream dress patterned with orange and brown flowers. Rooster escorted me to Vanilla Ice which used to be a fetish club where you could explore various aspects of fetish, by playing, or watching or just talking.

I was playing around with a few guys, teaching them, spanking them, but because I was in a dress I didn't feel like Princess Spider. I was in a bit of a quandary, asking myself, Who am I? What am I? And I just felt the night becoming more and more naughty. I didn't have any pussy worship or anything like that at the club, but I remember when I came back Rooster asked me to stand up against this diamond link fence – one of my fantasies – hitching my dress up so that my arse, knickers and stocking tops were showing. I beckoned him over. I was definitely Maria by then. Rooster fucked me against the fence but he became a bit panicky about how exposed we were so he dragged me into an alleyway and took me up against the wall. Afterwards he went home.

I stood there for a moment, feeling the night coalesce against my skin, and I felt myself changing again. I slipped on my gloves, re-entered the house, picked up my cane and went down to the dungeon.

He was still lying there. I took off my knickers and fucked him on the floor. And I told him he was not the first man I had had that evening.

PERMISSION TO SPEAK: Slave Rooster

'*If there's one thing I've taken away from our relationship it's spontaneity. Prior to meeting her I was not quite as relaxed a person. I come from a pretty structured background. And she helped to break that down a little. She's always teasing and having fun with you. She brought out a side of me, a playful side, that is still with me today.*

'It's given me a taste for things I never really knew before. She gave me a glimpse of something, sexually, that I probably won't experience again. Even the little details, such as body smell, are important to her. She wears a perfume called Noa that is exquisite when mingled with her own natural bodily scent. She knows that when you're wearing a blindfold or a hood that your sense of smell will be heightened. When she comes up to you and whispers in your ear, you get that smell and it's mind-blowing. It's a huge part of her power.

'I've met some interesting women in my time, but nobody like her. She is the single most extraordinary woman I've ever met and am ever likely to meet.'

There's someone else. Secret from everybody except Twin. She's his creation. Helga. His name for Maria when she is really naughty. And my word, do I mean naughty. He'll stick wooden spoons in me and make me wear ridiculously high-heeled red shoes and nothing else. He makes me stagger around in his flat doing menial chores. Me naked in high heels doesn't do anything for me but I suppose it works if you're into me.

Helga has to scrub the floor. I get given a little blue bowl and a yellow cloth and I have to crawl around in a load of slimy Cif and scrub the floor. The more I polish and get the floor wet, the more difficult it is to keep my balance. He'll tell me I'm giving him one of my views while I'm doing it and it's so humiliating. There's always candles, or low lighting, and some classical music in the background. We both like classical music. It's nice to slip into the rhythms and not be distracted by lyrics.

I do all that and he'll say, 'Helga, I think you need a shave,' so he'll get me on a towel on the sofa, not giving me a chance to clean up so I'm covered in soap suds and God knows what. And he'll spread my legs as wide apart as possible and cover me with baby oil and start shaving me. He'll get rid of it all or give me some designer style of his amusement. While he's shaving I might be forced to suck his cock.

Sometimes he likes to look as if he's not bothered by what's going on. So he'll smoke a cigarette and read the paper while I'm cleaning, as if to say, I don't give a fuck what you do. Or he might get me to masturbate and he'll go off to make a sandwich. He might have a peek now and again, but he doesn't need to watch me. I'll get foot worship but Helga has to wait for her punishment.

She has to kneel on the doormat and sometimes I'll be turned around so my bottom is exposed to him and he might approach and do something to it. One time he stroked me with this thing, I had no idea what it was, but it was glorious, all over my buttocks and cleft and back. I didn't know what it was until I saw him put it in his pocket and it turned out to be one of his sable oil painting brushes. It's so sexy. When he uses it on me it feels like I'm being painted.

Or he'll put me over the table with my legs apart and my arms splayed, blindfolded. And I'll wait there until he does something to me. I might be there for ages. I quite enjoy that because it's a very slow and drawn-out punishment. Although it's no punishment really. The punishment, as always, is not having punishment.

Later he'll drag me to the floor where he'll pull my hair, hauling me over to the sofa, where he'll bend me over, smother me with a handkerchief soaked in amyl nitrate, and fuck me like crazy.

Nobody else knows about Helga. It's Twin's little pleasure and nobody else's. I like it. It's another form of play for me. It doesn't bother me. He can do what he likes with me. I never feel threatened, just excited. I don't feel like an object.

When I first asked him to dominate me he was quite overawed because he was dating a famous mistress who was now asking him to beat her. But once we got over that little problem, everything was fine. I know he's seen a lot, done a lot. I wanted him to share some of his experiences, his knowledge with me. So I give him free rein when I'm in Helga mode. I'm his toy.

* * *

I have other identities I assume depending on the situation. It's important to have a portfolio of personalities; after all, we're playing a role more often than not. We have to earn our corn playing the part that our audience expects of us.

Some people want a medical session and on these occasions I will present a character known as Nurse Payne. Dumpling will come to me for a medical assessment. So I'll check that he's got a shaved cock and shaved balls. If he's a Body Slave I'll shave him completely down the middle of his bottom, so you've got skin touching skin instead of a buffer of hair. With a pair of tight pants it feels quite nice, apparently, until it starts to grow back.

Nurse Payne, resplendent in her blue nurse's uniform and surgical mask, gloves and thigh-high boots, will shave them with a Bic razor if they haven't done it. And then the tweezers come out for any errant hairs. You can't ignore the nipples. If they're clean shaven on the face there'll always be a few stragglers to attend to. Ears and noses might need trimming too. They might be tied down to a medical chair or bench while this is happening. I might incorporate nipple play with clamps and needles. If you pull the nipple out it's quite easy to push the needle straight through. When the needle is in you can twist it and pull it partially out to create different sensations.

And then there's the balls, of course, and the penis – all of it can have needles inserted, you just have to make sure the needles are sterile in their sealed packs, and they've been prepared with a sterile wipe beforehand. Needles are great because you can put them anywhere, and create patterns, you can even thread them with ribbon to create a bizarre body lacing effect on the back or chest. When it's done well it's very aesthetic.

Although it's a medical session there'll be some punishment involved too, so if they're wearing nipple clamps or needles, I'll probably flog them gently in those areas to generate some pain or discomfort. Or they could have a cock strap fitted with a spiked sheath. The spikes become more painful the more engorged the penis becomes. And of course there's the famous Wartenburg neurological pinwheel, which is nice over any part of the body.

I might put some headphones on them so they can hear one of my erotic stories while I torment them with needles. I might incorporate the electrical box; I'll strobe the violet wand anywhere below the waist.

It's completely different to a normal session. The setting is much more sterile and cold and clinical. You've got stainless steel shining all around you, all these weird and wonderful tools with blades and spikes and teeth that can be used on the flesh. Bright lights. The threat of anaesthetic and surgery. Slaves won't be begging in this scenario – well, maybe at the end – they just go in and sit down as if it's a dentist's chair. I like to wear a leather glove and a rubber glove while they're blindfolded so they think there are different hands working on them. Maybe they'll think another person has entered the operating theatre, and all well and good if they do. It gives them something else to think about and get nervous over.

You can use these big clamps on the nipples that are meant to stem bleeding during an operation. It's a great look to see these huge gleaming things hanging from a pair of nipples. Some of the other mistresses will take it further with catheters and enemas, but I never get guys asking for it so I don't do it. Some guys even like having their scrotum filled up with saline solution. You put a tube in once they've had a needle inserted and inject the saline so their balls become huge. I won't do that either, because of the risks involved. Some mistresses actually are nurses and will anaesthetise clients. Again, it's far too risky for me.

It's an extension of the dungeon scene. Ideally they won't just be fixated on that and we can spin things out to incorporate interrogation scenes, school sessions, foot worship. Medical sessions are special though, because you've got so much to play with and play around with their minds. They've seen all this equipment before they get their blindfolds on, so imagine what it must be like, lying there, immobile, and you hear the snap of latex as a glove goes on, or the clatter of a scalpel in a steel kidney-shaped bowl, or the hiss of gas from a mask.

These faces are there for whoever wants to see them: lover or slave, punter or confidante. What remains, though, despite the various facets of my life is my feeling for the people I am closest to. I love my slaves. When I'm with them, but not in session – perhaps we're at a club, or I've cooked for them, or they're doing a little job for me around the house – I feel totally at ease and natural with them. Some of them I'm happy to refer to as friends. I never feel I have to hide behind Princess Spider, or anybody else, when I'm with them.

Slave Daphne has seen me unwell; I have had problems with my back and leg. So he's seen me at my lowest ebb. All of them know I haven't been too well from time to time. They might see my vulnerable side, but they all love me in different ways precisely because they see I'm a normal person. Whatever 'normal' means …

One thing you should take away with you, especially if you're curious, or tempted: I don't play in the third week of every month because my PMT can cause me to be too vicious and I'd cut someone up badly! I might be in bad pain and I'd totally love it to destroy someone.

Keep in mind, then, that the first two weeks of my cycle are the best times to book an appointment with me…

It's getting dark. The city outside her window is steadily becoming bejewelled with lights from streetlamps, windows, cars nosing into or out of the urban sprawl. Think for a minute of all of the leaders and followers in those streets. Someone somewhere is always giving orders, taking orders. There are the powerful and the meek rubbing shoulders in bars and at bus stops. Dominants and submissives in every family, every office, every nook and cranny of this grand old town. In dungeons across London, across the world, men are kneeling before their mistresses, tensing their backs against the fire about to fall.

But not with the Princess. Not tonight. Her arms burn from the exertions of her last session; her voice is scratchy from all the shouting, commandments and withering put-downs. The Princess has luxuriated in a long hot bath. She has enjoyed a glass of fine wine. Now she lies in her bed, with its headboard of velvet, decked with the pegs and chains and straps of her mischief. She ignores the slaves texting and phoning her. This is her time. A time to refresh herself, replenish her energies. The night draws at her like an old friend but she resists it. It would be so easy to pull on the leather, the sunglasses, the spanking belt. It would be no trouble finding a cab to the club or the party. The friends would be there, the Body Slaves, the fans. Bottoms would be presented in the hope that the Princess might grant them a volley of slaps. But even the Spider must rest sometimes.

All the blood, sweat and tears that her torment has inspired, all the joy, laughter and ecstasy, all of it is forgotten now, at least for a little while. Sleep draws the Princess down into a world of shadow.

Who am I? What am I?

Inventive, feline, sensual, caring, inspiring. Dangerous when provoked. This deadly female of the species. Bittersweet threat. The Spider with a touch of velvet. Desire her, fear her; you can never ignore her.

She sleeps and the web of her dreams trembles with the breath of air as her victims approach, unable to resist.

Tomorrow she'll rise, reborn. Another glorious spectral return ...

SLAVE POWER BREAKDOWN

Princess Spider

Body Slave

Financial slave	Pain slave	Escort slave
Maid slave	Adult baby	Foot slave
Boot slave	Postal slave	Sissy slave
Text slave	Email slave	Phone slave
Slave in training	Scene slave	Newbie slave

*CONTRACT OF SLAVERY

I, known forever after always as Slave ....

Do hereby renounce my right of liberty and give myself freely and without reservation into the ownership of my Mistress,

PRINCESS SPIDER

I fully understand and accept the following conditions of my future existence as the slave of my Mistress:

- I am the property of my Mistress, body and mind.
- I will obey my Mistress at all times without question or hesitation.
- I accept that my feelings, opinions and wishes are meaningless and irrelevant.
- I will speak only when spoken to.
- I will kiss my Mistress's shoes, boots or feet as a greeting to her when and wherever I first meet her.
- I will always be naked in the presence of my Mistress or I will always dress up for an audience with Her in approved clothes.
- I will fully learn my duties as a slave to my Mistress.
- I am to accept fitting punishments for any behaviour unsuitable to a lowly slave.
- I accept that my body is useful only for the pleasure of my Mistress.
- I will accept any torture, punishment or humiliation my Mistress chooses for me.
- I will be completely honest about my fantasies and desires.
- I will confess any disobedience or failings and ask to be punished for them.
- During the course of my punishment I fully accept that I may be marked and that any punishment I may be given is my sole responsibility.

Signed (Mistress) ....

Signed (Slave) ....

Witnessed ....

Witnessed ....

Date ....

A typical slave contract. Original devised by Mistress Sidonia von Bork.

Princess Spider biography:

Based in London, Princess Spider is one of the most popular and respected Dominatrices in the UK and Europe. She writes for several magazines and websites, like *Massad*, *Tied and Teased* and *The London Fetish Scene*.

In 2004, she embarked on the successful and original television series 'Dominatrix Reloaded' for Granada/Sky Television. As well as writing and presenting the series, she co-produced the project for her Film and Television production company, Spifilms Ltd.

Her personal website can be found at www.princess-spider.com from which her monthly newsletter can be obtained. Princess Spider also creates Spider-related films, merchandise, CDs, phone games, phone services and original fetish music.